# Primary Care Trust Workforce
# Planning and Development

The software accompanying this book can be downloaded free of charge from www.healthcareworkforce.org.uk. If you have problems accessing the software then please e-mail the author: k.hurst@leeds.ac.uk

# Primary Care Trust Workforce Planning and Development

**KEITH HURST** PhD
Senior Lecturer,
Nuffield Health and Social Care Policy Group,
Health Sciences and Public Health Research Institute,
Leeds University

W
WHURR PUBLISHERS
LONDON AND PHILADELPHIA

© 2005 Whurr Publishers Ltd
First published 2005
by Whurr Publishers Ltd
19b Compton Terrace
London N1 2UN England and
325 Chestnut Street, Philadelphia PA 19106 USA

**British Library Cataloguing in Publication Data**

A catalogue record for this book
is available from the British Library.

ISBN 1 86156 487 2

# Contents

# Preface

Primary and community care managers face the same workforce planning and development challenges as their hospital counterparts. They wrestle with both sides of the workforce planning and development (WP&D) equation: what size and mix of staff are needed to meet the locality's demands on one side, and once recruited how are staff retained and developed on the other. However, one large difference between community and hospital managers' efforts is that the former do not have the breadth and depth of approaches open to hospital managers (80 methods and related data at the last count). Consequently, information and algorithms to help primary care trust (PCT) managers plan and develop their teams are lacking. Any PCT manager faced with historically-based establishments, which at best are irrational and at worst fail to meet the locality's demands and generate inequitable workloads, would be forgiven for thinking he or she was the workforce planner Cinderella. However, a glass slipper is to hand.

What compound PCT managers' problems are the NHS modernization programmes, which call for new ways of doing things (such as Evercare and Advanced Access), against which they are regularly assessed. Moreover, accounting for almost three-quarters of PCT expenditure, staffing is not cheap and mistakes are not only costly to rectify but also subject to the 'oil tanker syndrome' where the effect of reversing the ship's propellers takes a protracted length of time before the vessel decelerates. Additionally, some healthcare professionals know they are a scarce resource and can choose when and where to work. Unbalanced workforce planning generates a vicious cycle; rising demand from primary and community care patients increases the workload for an already stretched workforce suffering long-term vacancies (up to 14%). Little wonder that employees move on. Less anecdotally but equally sobering, trust managers in one of the author's fieldwork sites were replacing one in six staff each year, which was thought to be workload stress-related – hardly conducive to good quality and continuous patient care.

It's only fair, therefore, that PCT managers are given the tools do their job: so now the good news. Agencies supporting and guiding managers, such as the Department of Health (DH), Office for National Statistics

(ONS) and the Healthcare Commission, have systematically collected and summarized a comprehensive list of WP&D variables and data (90 at the latest count). Moreover, once permission to copy these variables and data is obtained (a straightforward process), WP&D variables and data are easily called up by computer. Users will notice that information is almost always organized by co-terminus PCT and Local Authority, incredible foresight for which someone deserves an award. Consequently, all the tumblers fall into place, opening a door to a WP&D solution-rich vault. One task remained, however, that of pulling together the PCT-based data from several agencies into one location, organizing them, and writing guidance material that 'walks' managers through the information and options.

Accompanying this book (the guide), therefore, is software (see later for the URL), which is the vault. Readers are introduced to the PCT WP&D software's nature and utility via a case study PCT. They should find it easy to replace the case study trust's data with their own and draw similar or different WP&D conclusions and recommendations. The software's structure means that managers can benchmark their locality's demographic, socio-economic, morbidity, mortality, activity, performance and staffing data with PCTs in the same socio-economic band. They also can compare their trust's state-of-play with 3-star PCTs while other, equally ingenious comparisons are possible.

Also included in this book is a detailed annotated bibliography dedicated to PCT WP&D. Publications are referenced in the usual way but additionally a précis is attached so that readers can judge the material's merits before following-up key issues at the source. The annotated bibliography uses key words such as community patient dependency. Consequently, readers should be able to capitalise on these three reserves. It is intended to keep the software fresh so that managers can access state-of-the-art information thereby extending the book's shelf life immeasurably.

Despite the composite PCT WP&D database's value, the variables' and data's implications can take time and effort to unravel. For example, should trust managers use the Census population or GP list size as the denominator for estimating the number of staff? Workshops, therefore, are being organized to help PCT managers explore the software and book. A helpline is also open for readers and software users (helpline and workshops are free and queries should be directed to the author using the e-mail address below). What only remains, therefore, is to wish readers successful forays into the world of primary and community WP&D.

Keith Hurst
Health Sciences and Public Health Research Institute, Leeds University
February 2005
k.hurst@leeds.ac.uk

# Acknowledgements

The Department of Health, Mansfield District and Nottingham City Primary Care Trusts and the NHS National Workforce Projects commissioned the studies. The author is grateful for the support and information provided by the DH, Office for National Statistics, Healthcare Commission (formerly the Commission for Health Improvement) and for their permission to use the data. Several other PCTs generously gave their time and resources. Thanks are due to my Leeds University academic colleagues: Justin Keen, Brenda Leese and Jackie Ford for reading and commenting on draft chapters. However, the book's conclusions and recommendations are the author's alone. Finally, I am grateful to my wife, Jean, for the inordinate time she spent helping me to locate and cross reference data that forms the software.

# CHAPTER ONE

# Introduction, background and context

There can be little doubt about the importance of National Health Service (NHS) workforce planning – especially staff demand and supply – not least because health and social services employ one in ten people from the UK working population and staff costs account for two-thirds of NHS expenditure (Kendall and Lissauer 2003). Although these data relate to the whole NHS, this book focuses on the primary and community-care workforce planning and development.

Primary care and community care are defined in many ways. Their main distinguishing features are the setting in which care is given and the professionals who provide the service. Primary care is the first-contact, continuous and coordinated care of individuals. Community care, on the other hand, is linked to a much wider social network. Primary and community care, therefore, are not synonymous with general practice, but they do subsume it (Mackenzie and Ross 1997). Consequently, primary care and community care are distinguished in this book because the service context influences workforce planning and development.

Primary and community care are said to have six cardinal principles (Department of Health or DoH 1993a, 1993b, 2000a, 2001a, 2002b; Hodder 1995; Richards et al. 2000; Hyde 2001):

1. Safe, effective, efficient, devolved, open and accountable community services.
2. Accessible and appropriate services designed to meet community and individual needs, which include a range of treatment choices.
3. Access to named, skilled practitioners.
4. Services that do not discriminate between any individual or group.
5. Twenty-four-hour seamless care among primary, community and secondary settings.
6. Owing to the remote and isolated working, good employment practices that, for example, minimize workplace violence.

The intention behind these six principles is to help vulnerable people live independently in their homes or other community settings. They should raise community patients' quality of life while at the same time reducing cost-ly, institutional care (Anonymous 1994). Maintaining these cardinal principles through efficient and effective community and primary care work-force planning and development have become a primary care trust (PCT) priority in recent months (DoH 2001a; Bosma and Higgins 2002; Tobin 2002).

## Workforce planning and development definitions

Initially, Department of Health policy documents indicated that primary and community care workforce planning and development were about predict-ing the future demand for different types of practitioners while seeking to match supply with the demand for staff. Later the Department of Health (DoH 2001a, p. 12, 2002b, para 1.2) presented a more sophisticated defini-tion of workforce planning and development:

> [workforce planning and development is a] dynamic process that aims to ensure PCTs have the right people with the right skills in the right place at the right time. This means the processes used to determine the workforce of today and the future needs to be a rigorous one, using knowledge held with-in an organisation supported by techniques that assess the future.

The premises on which the Department of Health's (2001a, p. 15) rationale for this definition are based are:

> Increasing the number of staff training for an NHS career is vital if we are to increase the capacity of the NHS and its ability to deliver faster and better care for patients. It is not by itself enough to deliver the increases in staff numbers we need, particularly in the short term. We shall, therefore, inten-sify our drive to attract people to healthcare careers, to retain them when they have joined the NHS and to encourage those who have left to return to practice, and we shall step up our plans for international recruitment to meet demands in the short term before an increased number of staff come through training.

The relationship between the demand for staff and their supply is under-lined in this quotation. An earlier Department of Health report (2000b) indicated a growing concern with NHS and higher education staff efforts to address workforce demand and supply. Workforce planning, the staff felt, should be embedded in the NHS culture which ought to lead to efficient and effective workforce planning and development. These are needed not only to reduce short-term staffing solutions but also to meet the demand for future health-care needs. Workforce planning and development can be represented as shown in Figure 1.1 (DoH 2000a).

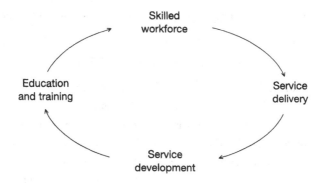

**Figure 1.1** Workforce planning and development.

# Driving and restraining forces

Without doubt primary and community care staff have an important NHS role. Despite their importance, historically, low levels of spending and understaffing (compared with Europe, for example) meant that too few workers struggled to provide care in challenging circumstances. Moreover, work pressures increased relentlessly and, coupled with a better informed and less deferential public, meant that practitioners faced even greater challenges (Kendall and Lissauer 2003). Researchers such as Lewis and deBene (1994) and Latimer and Ashburner (1997) believed that primary and community care success depended on services meeting the following challenges:

- Primary and community carers are capable of raising their contribution.
- Health services are based in the right care setting – caring rather than curing services are more appropriate in the community than in hospitals and community patients are capable of self-care. Similarly, health promotion is more suited to primary care.
- Increasing hospital throughput and transfer of services between health and social care mean that secondary care efficiency and effectiveness will suffer if primary and community care staff do not raise their game.
- The biomedical model alone cannot meet a modern primary and community care agenda.
- Learning about a population, especially inner cities, whose health needs are unmet.

One positive feature of recent health-care policy and practice developments is that, after years of chronic under-funding, resources are being moved from acute to primary and community care (Latimer and Ashburner 1997). Nevertheless, a number of driving and restraining forces govern PCT management and practice (DoH 2002b) (Table 1.1).

**Table 1.1** Driving and restraining forces that govern primary care trust management and practice

| Driving | Restraining |
| --- | --- |
| Increasing staff autonomy | Extended role limitations |
|  | Recruitment and retention |
| Prevention and caring as important as curing | Competing for resources |
| Hospital efficiency and effectiveness |  |
| Local population health-care needs | Inverse care law |
| Policy developments | Sparse workforce planning and development data and methods |
| Patient choice |  |
| Continuous quality improvement |  |
| New General Medical Service contract | Traditional professional groups |

PCT managers have varying degrees of control over these drivers. Moreover, only 9% of managers in a recent survey felt that their workforce planning and development efforts were supported by their superiors and subordinates (Bosma and Higgins 2002). One reason for the lack of support and confidence is that PCT managers, unlike their hospital counterparts, do not have the variety of methods for estimating appropriate size and mix of health-care teams that are available to their hospital counterparts (Hurst 2003). Most of the primary and community care workforce planning literature is anecdotal and only a handful of systematic, empirically determined methods are available (Syson-Nibbs 1997; Richards et al. 2000; Tobin 2002). In addition, few national community and primary staffing models exist and, of the broader ones out there, none accommodates the implications of recent policy and practice developments such as the following:

- National Service Frameworks (NSFs)
- Modernization programmes, such as the Changing Workforce Programme, which address pay, learning, personal development and professional regulation
- Liberating the Talents
- National Primary Care Development Team initiatives
- New General Medical Service contract and Personal Medical Service pilots.

These more recent policy and practice initiatives are guaranteed to shape the future primary and community care workforce (Buchan and Edwards

2000; DoH 2002b, 2002c; NHS Workforce Taskforce et al. 2002) because of the following:

- Widening patient choice
- Strengthening patient voices
- Local strategies for tackling inequalities
- The availability of round-the-clock primary and community care
- Ageing population and increasing chronic illness
- Improving interfaces between primary and secondary care
- Increasing secondary care in the community
- Increasingly technological care and service innovations such as NHS Direct and walk-in centres
- One-service approach to health and social care
- Re-designing roles and tasks and broadening staff mix
- Extending practitioner roles
- Strengthened leadership at the coalface
- Focusing on prevention.

Clearly, future workforce planning and development endeavours in the primary and community care sectors have to address a range of management and clinical issues.

## Workforce planning and development method issues

Different workforce planning and development needs and approaches make it difficult for managers to look across primary and secondary care settings in a uniform way. Moreover, people's need for care is not always neatly divided into primary and secondary care domains, and staff should not be categorized in this way either. Unfortunately, this may mean that fragmented and uniprofessional approaches to workforce planning and development remain despite recent attempts to improve integration. Dissonance is heightened when Department of Health policy makers (2000a, 2002c) believed that primary and community care workforce planning:

- failed to build research and development into planning, although, as we shall see later, the breadth and depth of workforce-related data are strong, there is a shortage of empirically determined techniques for modelling them
- has inconsistent focus on staff mix
- managers were not motivated to improve their strategies until recent health policy documents and guidance emerged and, consequently, a willingness to change followed.

Recent major policies such as *Liberating the Talents* (DoH 2002c) try to encapsulate workforce planning driving and restraining issues, and integrate planning and development, within three new categories of work:

1. First contact: acute assessment, diagnosis, treatment, care and referral.
2. Continuing care: NSF-oriented rehabilitation and chronic disease management.
3. Public health: promotion and protection that improve health and reduce inequalities.

Implementation of this framework may give PCT managers an even greater workforce planning and development challenge because specific data tend to be organized along traditional workforce lines, i.e. health visiting, district nursing, community therapists, etc. Currently, the literature reveals four broad primary and community care workforce planning and development categories:

1. Professional judgement or manager–practitioner consensus approaches
2. Population and health needs based
3. Caseload analysis
4. Acuity or workload methods that use patient classification and activity times.

The first method, professionally judging the level of staffing in the context of safety and quality of primary and community care, is identical to the inpatient counterpart of the same name (Waite 1986). A team of locally knowledgeable managers and practitioners decide a care team's size and mix. The method is quick and inexpensive but results are often labelled subjective because there are few empirical underpinnings. The second method, health needs analysis, uses:

- demographic and biographic variables such as population density and age (Coffey undated; Piggott 1988; DoH 2002a)
- socioeconomic data such as deprivation and housing (Piggott 1988; Ebeid 2000)
- morbidity and mortality data such as General Health Questionnaire (GHQ) scores (Durrand 1989).

These variables and data provide a good base from which to determine the size and mix of teams. Obviously, to make this approach workable, staffing ratios such as the number of district nurses per head of population are also required. The method's value lies in its staffing algorithms which reflect, for example, a locality's deprivation or geographical spread. In later chapters, relevant data for each PCT are provided for the reader.

The third or caseload analysis method, which includes data such as the number of contacts, is another important and useful approach to estimating the size and mix of care teams (Waite 1986; Luft 1990; Frame and O'Donnell 1996). However, merely attaching care times to activities and using the results are not enough (Coffey, undated). Drennan (1990a) explains how invaluable dependency and workload data can be. Later, however, she showed that similar-sized caseloads did not always generate the same amount of work, i.e. caseload size did not always equate to workload (Drennan 1990b). Moreover, Buchan (1999) explained how stress-related job dissatisfaction is influenced by workload, which implies that getting caseload right is imperative in these days of staff and skills shortage. In short, these data are also useful for improving recruitment and retention.

Several authors indicate the information needed for caseload analysis although information will vary depending on the professional group (Dobby and Barnes 1987a; Barret and Hudson 1997; Audit Commission 1999; Dewis 2001):

- service objectives and referral criteria
- new referral numbers
- number and type of assessments and reassessments
- essential and non-essential work
- community patient age distribution
- direct and indirect care
- clerical and administrative work
- travelling
- time spent on the practitioner's caseload.

Dewis (2001) recommended that model caseloads be built from these data before practice teams are benchmarked against them. Once these data are available, it just remains either to modify policies and procedures or to make staffing adjustments. Consequently, another important application of the caseload approach is to modify a practitioner's workload to establish equity as well as reviewing the number and mix of staff.

There is overlap between the caseload analysis approach and the fourth workforce-planning category – the dependency–acuity method. The latter, however, aggregates data from a number of localities (Audit Commission 1999). Goldstone et al. (2000) developed and tested the dependency–acuity method extensively in the community, which Goldstone and his colleagues had started 20 years earlier (Goldstone and Worrall 1980). They concluded that two systematically collected data-sets – patient characteristics and staff activity – help primary and community care managers.

The dependency–acuity protocol is clear and logical:

- Each patient is assigned to a dependency group that ranges from one (minimum) to four (maximum reliance on carers).
- To accommodate domestic variables, weighting is added to the dependency scores for community patients with below-average family support.

Dependency and the corresponding amount of nursing effort (in minutes) are entered into a simple algorithm given in Goldstone et al. (2000). The advantage of community dependency–acuity systems is that they offer a standardized approach that avoids duplicating effort in other PCTs. The validity and reliability of instruments can easily be tested (compared with, for example, health needs assessment measures). Consequently, the outcomes are operationally and strategically valuable data (Drennan 1990b; Goldstone et al. 2000).

Unlike hospitals, the community is never 'full', which makes workload measures even more important to ensure workload equity. Consequently, primary and community care dependency–acuity data have several valuable functions (Coffey, undated; Fitton 1984b; Luft 1990; Frame and O'Donnell 1996):

- Tracking and comparing dependency and workload over time and between areas
- Equalizing, rationalizing and prioritizing work
- Highlighting mismatches between ideal and actual staffing
- Indicating informal carers' contribution to patient care
- Encouraging a common language between commissioners and practitioners
- Assisting decision-making about the size and mix of community teams
- Informing joint working with social services.

Dewis (2001) criticizes the primary and community workforce-planning armoury because:

- retrospective and aggregated data are less valuable
- dependency ratings can be subjective and inflated
- non-standard community patient dependency scoring systems are used
- data processing errors are not uncommon.

Given the lack of consensus and workforce planning and development's controversial nature, a multifaceted approach ought to be used.

# This book's aim, objectives and methods

Hospital workforce planning methods, despite their breadth, depth and power, do not translate into community and primary care settings. The main reason is that patient dependency and face-to-face activity, as the two main community workload variables, can be overwhelmed by, for example, the travelling that practitioners undertake between patients' homes (Coffey undated) and the likelihood that patients may not be at home, i.e. inpatient-staffing formulae are more sensitive to 'direct patient care' than 'associated work' such as travel, which make inpatient methods inappropriate for estimating the number of primary and community care staff. On the positive side, the author's literature review unearthed a wealth of material that is relevant and important to community and primary care workforce planning (see Annotated bibliography, page 167). In short, several community and primary care workforce planning and development issues and challenges emerge from the literature (DoH 1998, 2001a, 2002b; Bosma and Higgins 2002):

- A deliberate intention to increase the number of primary and community practitioners substantially.
- Efficient and effective local workforce planning that creates a modern workforce, which not only meets patients' needs but also develops services and improves their efficiency and effectiveness.
- Evaluating and investing in the local workforce to reduce attrition and to develop staff with the capacity, skills, diversity and flexibility to meet changing and rising service demands.
- Managers and practitioners, who are able to exploit information and technology, and thereby increase service efficiency and effectiveness.
- Forming partnerships with education, social care and other agencies to increase workforce planning efficiency and effectiveness that meets and capitalizes on the rising number of training places.
- Developing managers' workforce planning knowledge and skills to help them address gloomy but inescapable workforce predictions and break down professional barriers that restrict the way practitioners work.
- Building and using robust databases generally for demand-side primary and community care workforce planning, and specifically for the changing workforce programme.

To meet these challenges, and especially to make workforce planning more sensitive to primary and community care, PCT workforce planners are expected to do at least the following (DoH 2001a, 2002b):

- Identify future demand for primary and community services. An area of high deprivation will, for example, require a different set of practitioner knowledge skills from an affluent area. Recognize the different demands that these areas throw up, planning and developing the workforce accordingly.

- Map the existing workforce.
- Identify the gaps between workforce size and mix and the health needs analysis.
- Write and implement local workforce plans.

Given these issues, coupled with some pressing local staffing matters such as NSF and NHS modernization programme expectations, a detailed and extensive workforce planning and development study was implemented with the twin aims of:

1. collating and summarizing national and local data to inform primary and community care workforce planning and development
2. providing manual and computer-based algorithms to help managers determine ideal short- and long-term staffing.

As raised earlier, the paucity of community and primary demand-side workforce methods and related data are major barriers to effective PCT strategic and operational management, e.g. Buchan and Edwards (2000) warn managers using professional judgement methods alone that they may under- or over-estimate the size and mix of health-care teams. A triangulation approach is therefore used in this book to meet the project's two main aims. Consequently, the objectives and related methods include:

1. Black and Hagel's (1996) and Goodwin's (1994) suggestion that robust health needs assessment data are important for several reasons, including workforce planning and development. Consequently, the Department of Health, Office for National Statistics (ONS) Census 2001, Healthcare Commission (formerly the Commission for Health Improvement or CHI) and local PCT databases were interrogated. Data relating to about 90 demographic, socioeconomic, morbidity, mortality, personnel and performance variables (described in detail later), felt to influence the size and mix of primary/community teams, were attached to PCTs. These variables can be thought of as:

   – structure, such as staff:population ratios
   – process, such as the number of contacts per practitioner
   – output and outcomes, such as immunization rates.

2. Information from the synthesized database is used mainly to benchmark PCTs and recommend staff numbers and mix under various conditions such as areas with high deprivation, etc. In short, important variables such as PCT populations are used to estimate the number and mix of primary and community care staff in this report.

3. Individual interviews were conducted with several PCT managers. Discussions centred on interviewees' perceptions of their actual and ideal workforce size and mix. National and local policy and practice, and their influence on workforce planning and development, were also considered during the interviews. This qualitative component added local intelligence to the project that would have been impossible to generate from other sources.

4. As might be expected, data from objectives 1–3 were compared and contrasted with similar issues emerging from a deep and wide literature search (500 articles, books and reports to date, see Annotated bibliography, page 167).

The Department of Health, Office for National Statistics and Healthcare Commission databases were trawled for workforce-related variables and data, and organized into a PCT workforce planning and development (WP&D) database (how this was achieved is shown in Table 1.2).

Table 1.2 PCT workforce planning and development (WP&D) structure

| Variables | Structure | Grouped results |
|---|---|---|
| 15: demographic, e.g. age } | | {Deprived areas |
| 14: morbidity/mortality, e.g. CHD } | | {ONS Bands 1–6 |
| 14: socioeconomic, e.g. lone parents} | 304 PCTs | {Productivity |
| 28: performance, e.g. GP access } | | {Staff mix, etc. |
| 19: staffing, e.g. nurses per capita } | | {CHI star ratings |

CHD, coronary heart disease; CHI, Commission for Health Improvement.
Permission to use the data for the information on PCT WP&D database is greatly appreciated.

Variables and related data have been aligned to each PCT and tagged, among other things, with a Healthcare Commission star rating and an ONS socioeconomic band. Consequently, not only has each of the 304 English PCTs been profiled in the PCT WP&D database but each has also been benchmarked in several ways:

- The database, available from www.healthcareworkforce.org.uk allows the reader to rank his or her PCT in a 'league table' of 304 trusts. Examples and detailed analyses are given in later chapters.
- The reader can also benchmark his or her PCT with trusts in the same ONS Band, e.g. one specimen PCT used in this book is in ONS Band 6, along with 82 other trusts, so case study PCT data are compared with structures, processes and outcomes emerging only from ONS Band 6 PCTs.

There are six ONS Bands:

ONS 1: inner city
ONS 2: port, mining and industrial towns
ONS 3: mixed economy urban centres
ONS 4: service, education, resort and retirement areas
ONS 5: prosperous and growth centres
ONS 6: mixed urban, rural or coast locations.

Banding is important because it would be unfair and inaccurate to compare ONS Band 1 data with ONS Band 6 PCTs. Finally, average values from 43 three-star PCTs are also provided against which the reader can compare his or her trust.

## Conclusion

Good quality primary care and community care help patients to live independently in the community, raise quality of life and improve service efficiency and effectiveness. Appropriate size and mix of primary and community health-care teams are a fundamental requirement for these outcomes. Notwithstanding the growing demand for primary and community services as the population changes and services move from hospital to community, PCT managers face several challenges such as implementing new policies. Other issues in the literature that drive and restrain PCT WP&D are lucid and compelling, which leave PCT managers in no doubt about what is expected of them if primary and community care are to succeed and secondary care is not hindered.

Primary and community care WP&D definitions and models in the literature are logical and clear. They are about getting enough practitioners with the right skills not only to meet primary and community health-care demands but also to develop and implement new services. However, unlike their hospital counterparts, PCT managers do not have the breadth and depth of methods or data to help them plan and develop their workforce. At least three problems emerge from longstanding primary and community care methods. First, there is a risk that primary and community care WP&D will be fragmented and unidisciplinary when modern workforce planning should concentrate on integrated working. Second, and related to this, policies such as *Liberating the Talents* focus on patients' needs, which call for competency and protocol-based workforce decisions. Third, recruitment and retention supply-side problems can easily stymie managers' best endeavours. However, appropriately triangulated demand-side methods can help managers make workloads equitable among disparate groups and isolated practitioners – an important job satisfaction and staff retention issue. It seems vital that PCT managers be given robust data and algorithms – the main aim of this text.

# CHAPTER TWO

# Community patient dependency and workload

## Introduction and background

Community dependency relates to patient demands for personal, technical and supportive care and education, which strongly influence primary and community practitioners' workloads (Durrand 1989). As raised in Chapter 1, measurement of community patient dependency, workload and corresponding staffing requires different approaches to those used in hospitals (Prideaux 1996).

As readers may have noticed, the literature covering primary and community care dependency and workload can seem contradictory and unhelpful. Moreover, a surprising number of authors such as Gibbing (1995) and Ross (1980b) are antagonistic towards measuring community patient dependency, especially using unmodified activities-of-living-based instruments, which are a strong feature of inpatient workforce planning methods. There is also a warning in the literature that measuring methods should not add to practitioners' burdens because the primary and community care administrative workload is rising anyway (Luft 1990). Goodman's (1996) and Crofts et al.'s (2000) studies showed that community nurses regard information collection negatively. Several reasons for these perceptions were noted either in the literature or during interviews with primary care trust (PCT) managers:

- Nineteen per cent of community nurses' caseloads include patients who have been 'on the books' for 5 years or more (Drennan 1990a).
- Data collection instruments had low validity and reliability and forms failed to articulate adequately the complex nature of primary and community care as a result of practitioners' day-to-day problem-solving and decision-making experiences.
- Correlation between a community patient's health needs and workload measures seems weak.
- Admitting partial responsibility, practitioners said that they coped with rising workloads by reorganizing care and not by systematically recording the change and underlying reasons when the size and mix of community teams were inadequate.

Consequently, routine dependency and activity data collection and recording were seen as a burden that had little benefit at the 'coalface'. On the other hand, when evaluating nursing teams, Barriball and Mackenzie (1993) felt that it was not enough for practitioners to act only as sources of information. They must also interpret the data that they collect and use the results to guide practice and to demonstrate efficiency and effectiveness. Billingham (1991) admitted that health needs assessment, an important proxy measure of dependency and workload, is complex. Mackenzie and Ross (1997), on the other hand, felt that community nurse research and development knowledge and skills needed developing even if workload pressures were eased so that time was made for collecting and interpreting information. Ideally, therefore, PCT managers should not add to community practitioners' administrative burden, but they should try to use existing data and involve practitioners in their interpretation and application.

Nevertheless, there are distinct benefits to caseload profiling and health needs assessment:

• discharging patients to more appropriate services
• monitoring caseloads
• workload measurement and achieving equitable case mixes
• shaping care programmes
• formulating competencies
• contributing to discussions with commissioners.

As the Audit Commission (1999) noted, however, few patient dependency and nursing workload algorithms and benchmarks can be found in the literature. This may explain why more than half of the community practitioners in the Audit Commission's (1999) study were not involved in health needs assessment or caseload profiling. This seems odd because Colliety (1988b), Crofts et al. (2000) and Mackenzie and Ross (1997) noted that community nurses understand local health needs as well any health-care professional. Consequently, there is concern that their knowledge and data are not fully used. These problems are compounded because extraction of health needs information is difficult as a result of the narrative form. Crofts et al. (2000), on the other hand, saw qualitative data as a solution to substandard data-sets because of their richness.

Another problem, an acute one occurring in the present study, was that health and local authority boundaries are not always co-terminus. Therefore data collected by one agency cannot always be equated to a relevant health district. Drennan (1990a) pointed out that co-terminus boundaries greatly assist workload assessment, workforce planning and development, not least because connections can be made between health and social care. Triggle (2003) explored co-terminosity from another perspective: he noted that local authority and health authority managers disagreed on the most important and useful data-sets. Deprivation, cancer and circulatory diseases were universally rated highly, but managers parted on the importance of teenage pregnancy, substance abuse, unemployment, fragmented communities, smoking and mental health. These issues are important because Roberts and Anstead (1996) showed how collaboration between health and social care managers encouraged multi-agency working that led to better resource use.

Some of the problems highlighted so far may explain why manager interviewees were only able to restrict referrals rather than strategically plan patient care in relation to practitioners' caseloads – crisis management in short. Trust managers, with or without co-terminus data, need to know the demand for community care so that services are based on need and staff being deployed efficiently and effectively (Audit Commission 1994, 1999; Mackenzie and Ross (1997). Goodwin (1994, p. 128) explains:

> In the primary health care setting it is difficult to see how anything rational could be done to adjust [staff mix] without having first undertaken a systematic practice population, neighbourhood and caseload health profiling exercise involving all members of the team, in order to identify the amount and type of care needed and, indeed to inform the purchasing strategy and contracting more generally . . . . Practice profiles compiled by health visitors and district nurses [for example] are being used to . . . plan staffing levels; all of which address concerns about efficiency and effectiveness.

Goodwin (1994) was worried that without services based on community patient needs there is a risk that commissioners will increase the numbers of lower-grade staff to save money.

## Dependency measures

Ong (1991) found it difficult not only to determine specific categories of patient need but also to match them with workload. She felt that the diffuse nature of community patients' needs and the way patients straddle community and Social Service boundaries was partly to blame. Nevertheless, Ong identified three types of patients and carers that influence community practitioners' work. Generally, patients:

- saw themselves as people rather than diseases and were clear about practitioners' roles
- regarded their illness as a discrete episode, tried to limit its impact and perceived clear boundaries between independence and reliance on professionals

- do not distinguish between them and their illness and expect practitioners to see the totality of their needs.

Ong (1991) classified carers as:

- engulfed in the caring role, unable to distinguish between their and the patients' needs
- fulfilled by a caring role, failing to recognize their needs and who may resist assistance
- boundary setters who underline the difference between their and the patients' needs and distinguish practitioners' prerogatives accordingly.

Ong's analysis underlines the theoretical and practical issues surrounding community patient classification. In view of dependency and workload data's complexity and importance, several patient dependency-rating instruments were explored by the author. Poulton (1984), for example, used a patient-dependency score based on the Crichton Royal Behavioural Rating Scale whereas Dobby and Barnes (1987a) classified patients using a combination of physical, psychological and social needs and the probable help required. The North American Kaiser Permanente community patient dependency levels also offer another simple but useful workload assessment instrument (Craig 2003):

Level 3:  intensive, coordinated, optimized care
Level 2:  short-term assisted care for self-help patients
Level 1:  routine care needing period assessment, monitoring clinical management, education and social support.

Between 70% and 80% of Kaiser Permanente North American community patients were level 1. Daubert (1979), another North American researcher, devised an unusual patient classification system based on aims and objectives that professionals, patients and carers are expected to achieve:

Group 1: non-chronic episodic disease or disability where the patient is expected to return to pre-illness health. This aim has three objectives and supporting criteria.
Group 2: chronic illness patient experiencing an acute episode but who is likely to revert to pre-exacerbation state; supported by six objectives and criteria.
Group 3: patient suffering a chronic illness with a possibility of reverting to the former episodic state. There are nine supporting objectives and criteria.
Group 4: a chronically ill patient who can be maintained at home without home care services. There are 10 objectives and criteria.
Group 5: end-stage illness category with 11 objectives and criteria.

These groups, supporting objectives and criteria have the advantage of:

- obviating the need to write a care plan
- saving time writing a discharge form
- serving as outcome measures that are useful for addressing the reasons for efficiency, effectiveness, service success rate and failures
- helping managers to estimate staffing needs; caseloads with predominantly group 4 and 5 patients need not only more staff but also practitioners with different skills
- helping managers to cost their service.

Townsend's (Williams et al. 1992) UK-oriented dependency scale, regularly encountered in the literature, has stood the test of time. Community patients are assessed on eight activities-of-living criteria:

1. walking up and down stairs
2. catching a bus
3. going shopping and carrying heavy bags
4. preparing and cooking hot meals
5. removing objects from overhead shelves
6. knot tying
7. cutting own toe nails
8. bathing or washing all over.

Ross's (1980b) work with rating instruments similar to Townsend's (Williams et al. 1992) showed that 66% of her community patients were capable of self-care and, of the remaining 34%:

- 17% needed help walking
- 6% were chair fast
- 12% were bed ridden.

Crofts et al.'s (2000) three-group classification in the UK showed that 36% of community patients fell into the lowest dependency level. The Audit Commission (1999) noted that 85% of district nurses' patients were low dependency and one in ten scored the lowest possible rating.

Malone and Mackenzie (2000) divided their patients into groups with particular problems. These are compared with Drennan's (1990a) typologies in Table 2.1. These data underline the data consistency problems that primary and community care managers face.

Shepherd (1992) devised a community child patient dependency instrument based on an ill-health risk scale. The scale included 26 health factors, which indicated a long-term health risk. These factors were socioeconomic, lifestyle or morbidity related, and were scored using a scale that ranged from 'factor present but no effect on children' to 'immediate effect on a child's

**Table 2.1** Groups of patients with particular problems

| Dependency criteria | Malone and Mackenzie (2000) (%) | Drennan (1990a) (%) |
|---|---|---|
| Depression | 40 | |
| Confusion | 88 | |
| Aggression | 31 | |
| Incontinence | 68 | |
| Needing supervision | 48 | 40 |
| Frail companion | | 11 |
| Supported accommodation | | 5 |
| Pastoral care | 70 | |
| Communication problems | 50 | 15 |
| Pressure sore risk | 44 | |
| Help with nutrition | 25 | |
| Ethnic minorities | | 18 |

health'. One family in six from Shepherd's study scored significantly on the health risk scale:

- 63% were lone parents of whom half were younger than 21 years
- almost all were benefit dependent
- three-quarters smoked and 10% abused alcohol
- a quarter had a history of mental illness and the same proportion had been the victim of violence.

Shepherd's work seems particularly relevant to health visiting and school nursing. Elsewhere, health visitors have adopted the Registrar General's social classes I–V to prioritize their work (Reading and Allen 1997).

The variation in community patient dependency data noted during the author's systematic review of the literature could be genuine or it may be that instruments' psychometric properties (such as inter-rater reliability) are suspect. Although these data are invaluable for determining staff mix, they vary over time and from place to place although, meta-analytically, the literature suggests that the bulk of community practitioners' caseload consists of low-dependency patients.

# Dependency and workload

The interrelationship of community practitioner staffing, activity, dependency and workload is complex. The Audit Commission (1999) are among many who warned that community staff activity may not be an accurate measure of workload. Nevertheless, serious attempts have been made to create instruments that indicate not only patient dependency but also the workload generated, e.g. Tieisinga et al. (1994), using regression analysis, showed that patient dependency was a good predictor not only of basic care but also of technical care workload. Similarly, Prideaux (1996) seemed confident about assessing community workload from the number of nursing interventions required by each patient.

One instrument for quantifying community patient dependency and workload using a combination of materials from the literature and expert professional views was used by the author in the present study. In practice, practitioners were asked to rate current patients using a combination of patient dependency and nursing effort ratings (available from the author at k.hurst@leeds.ac.uk). Three dependency and workload levels were generated from an analysis of 378 patients in two PCTs (Table 2.2).

**Table 2.2** Analysis of patients in two primary care trusts

| Level | Score |
| --- | --- |
| Low dependency and workload | < 0.3 |
| Medium | 0.3–5.2 |
| High | > 5.2 |

In short, up to two-thirds of community patients generated workloads between 0.5 and 3.5 – the medium workload category. These data were a snapshot and, unfortunately, cannot be benchmarked more widely. However, although dated, Hudson and Hawthorn's (1989) survey showed a similar distribution.

Rookes (1982) devised a similar points system to indicate light and heavy health visiting workloads:

- children under 5 years
- dependent families
- over-65s
- physically and mentally disabled
- practice list size
- number of clinics
- day nursery and child minder visits
- fieldwork teacher responsibilities.

Four outcomes emerged:

1. A workload factor for each health visitor
2. Separate clinic workload indicators
3. Group workload indicators
4. Percentage of time spent on key activities.

Rookes' article also included a simple but valuable algorithm for converting dependency and workload data into ideal staff numbers. Reading and Allen (1997) determined health visiting workload from caseload analysis. Time spent on the following activities was important:

- Parenting programmes
- Postnatal support groups and breast-fed babies
- Low-birthweight babies and children with developmental problems
- Special behaviour clinics
- Community development
- Total number of families, births and pre-school children
- Single or teenage parents
- Homeless individuals.

Unplanned work, such as child protection, was excluded.

One outcome from the author's review was that, if dependency and workload rating instrument psychometric properties are robust, the data they generate can be informative, e.g. Richards et al. (2000) estimated that primary care workload has increased by the equivalent of 187 GPs in the last decade. Although no estimates are given for other members of the primary and community care team, their workloads are judged to have increased in line. The extent of rises in workload meant that 61–65% of community practitioners in Jenkins-Clarke and Carr-Hill's (2001) study worked excessive hours. Moreover, the authors suggested that consultations for minor health issues are likely to increase by 11 million in the next 20 years, which will probably fall into primary/community practitioners' remits. This change influences decisions about the number of 'first contact' staff needed in primary, community and secondary care. However, the broader picture is less clear because the number of community patient contacts, as discussed later, is falling yearly.

The choice and advice about using community patient dependency and workload measures may seem bewildering and off-putting. These criticisms may explain why some PCT managers have turned to proxy measures of community patient dependency and workload such as health needs assessment data.

## Health needs assessment and community profiling

Barriball and Mackenzie (1993) and the *Saving Lives* (Department of Health or DoH 1999c) report not only set targets for reducing health inequalities but also underline the importance of social, economic, environmental, health and well-being factors as important determinants of good and poor health. Indeed, these data are deemed vital to primary and community workforce planning and are often treated as proxy dependency and workload measures. Drennan (1990a, 1990b), Hyde (2001), the Royal College of Nursing (RCN 1993b, 1994) and Roberts and Anstead (1996) list the variables and related data needed for profiling-based dependency and workload measurement, and related workforce planning and development:

- population size and geographical characteristics
- age, sex and ethnicity
- languages
- disease, disability and employment
- housing and finance
- frailty
- carers including one-parent families
- mental and emotional state
- dependency on carers and family support
- complex care needs
- inpatient history
- new and follow-up patient visit ratios
- staffing characteristics and any unusual commitments
- recruitment and retention
- practitioners' concerns
- traffic congestion, mileage, travelling time and access to services
- service uptake such as immunization
- patient expectation and satisfaction.

Hyde (2001) and Lewis and deBene (1994) suggest that assessors answer a number of questions before profiling their local community:

- Is the principal concern health or social care, e.g. is housing a major problem?
- Is the assessment about populations or individuals, e.g. are minority groups an issue?
- Are scarce resources the main issue?
- Is the exercise about priority setting?
- Is the assessment explorative or definitive, e.g. are undefined health needs a worry?
- Is determining the most important needs expert led or do processes involve patients and carers?
- Are there issues between primary and secondary care services?

Depending on answers to these questions, it is likely that the profiler will use either a medical model or a socioeconomic-oriented assessment. The former differs from the latter in the following ways (Hyde 2001):

- Needs are measured using disease patterns, prevalence and incidence, including standardized mortality rates and finished consultant episodes.

- Identifying the people affected and where they live.
- When diseases peak.

But Hyde (2001) warns that medical model-driven profiles can lead to wrong foci if the impact of health interventions is considered rather than health needs, particularly deprivation and social exclusion. Consequently, Hyde (2001) and Plews et al.'s (2000) recommendations build the profile systematically using three phases.

*Phase 1*

1. Agree the health needs assessment aims and time scale
2. Mark out the population and its boundaries
3. Examine routine data from different sources
4. Prioritize areas needing in-depth analysis
5. Summarize the resources available for service changes.

*Phase 2*

1. Involve professionals and users
2. Decide which other agencies need to be involved.

*Phase 3*

1. Recommend evidence-based changes
2. Agree who can best implement the changes.

Done well, health needs assessment profiles help managers and practitioners (Hyde 2001):

- respond to health needs rather than reacting to demands
- prioritize needs, health and social services in the context of limited resources
- highlight service irregularities
- underline unmet needs and ways of addressing them
- combine users' and professionals' views
- describe and benchmark health and disease issues
- identify services from which people benefit
- use resources efficiently and effectively
- address clinical, ethical and economic considerations
- highlight research and development priorities.

However, Plews et al. (2000) list the barriers that profilers face:

- contracting mechanisms that are not conducive to public health work
- restrictive professional boundaries that discourage collaboration
- disinterested health-care professionals

- lack of managerial vision and leadership
- medical-model dominance and less importance placed on socioeconomic issues, thereby discouraging interprofessional collaboration.

However, recently introduced policies such as *Liberating the Talents* (DoH 2002c) may help managers and practitioners to overcome these problems.

Profiling seems a tall order but PCTs' standing in demographic, socio-economic, morbidity and mortality, productivity and performance league tables, selected for their insights into community patient dependency and workload, can be collated and analysed relatively easily. The PCT used as a case study in the remainder of this chapter helps readers to envisage a rounder dependency and workload picture. In Tables 2.3–2.14, mean values and percentiles for England are given along with the average value from PCTs that sit in the same Office for National Statistics (ONS) category band:

ONS Band 1: inner city (10 PCTs)
ONS Band 2: port or mining industrial towns (47 PCTs)
ONS Band 3: urban centres with mixed economies (37 PCTs)
ONS Band 4: service, education, resort and retirement areas (42 PCTs)
ONS Band 5: prosperous and growing (85 PCTs)
ONS Band 6: mixed urban, rural and coast locations (83 PCTs).

It seems fairer to compare a PCT with its ONS compatriots. For broader benchmarking purposes the percentiles in Tables 2.3–2.14 help the reader to place his or her PCT in a league table. The three-star PCT averages are shown separately and it is assumed that these top-rated PCTs have a majority of efficient and effective structures and processes, which provide an additional benchmark. The reader can download his or her PCT's profile from www.healthcareworkforce.org.uk before substituting his or her PCT's data in Tables 2.3–2.14.

# Demographic data

Broad demographic data are a good place for workforce planners to start profiling the PCT. To reiterate, Tables 2.3–2.14 have five main features. Row 1 gives the English average. The mean values from three-star PCTs are in row 2, which provide another benchmark. All six ONS band data provide appropriate benchmarks in rows 3a–3f and finally the specimen case study PCT value is shown along with the percentiles in which it sits. Our case study PCT's population growth is above average and greater than its Band 3 compatriots. Its population is much more crowded so it is likely that practitioners' travelling time (outside peak times) is lower. Ethnicity (the

**Table 2.3** Basic demographics

| Primary care trust | Growth (%) | Density (persons per square mile) | Ethnicity (%) |
|---|---|---|---|
| 1 England | +0.15 | 2427 | 7 |
| 2 Three-star PCTs | +0.08 | 2494 | 4 |
| 3a ONS Band 1 PCTs | +0.63 | 11 247 | 48 |
| 3b ONS Band 2 | +0.06 | 3980 | 3 |
| 3c ONS Band 3 | +0.15 | 5987 | 13 |
| 3d ONS Band 4 | +0.12 | 2687 | 6 |
| 3e ONS Band 5 | +0.31 | 1828 | 8 |
| 3f ONS Band 6 | +0.03 | 1224 | 3 |
| 4a Specimen Band 3 PCT | +0.19 | 8892 | 19 |
| 4b PCT's percentile | 58th | 85th | 18th |

proportion of black, Asian and other minority ethnic group people) in our specimen PCT is well above average. Interestingly, three-star PCTs (row 2) have a stable population, which is not only predominantly white but also sparsely crowded.

# Age groups and sex

One purpose of recent health and social care legislation was to allow vulnerable people to live as independently as possible in their own homes (Anonymous 1994), no easy task when demographic data show that the proportion of 65+ year olds in trust populations varies greatly (Table 2.4).

**Table 2.4** Age-related demographic data

| PCT/Band | < 6 years (%) | 6–15 years (%) | 16–24 years (%) | 25–64 years (%) | > 64 years (%) | Mean (years) | Female (%) |
|---|---|---|---|---|---|---|---|
| England | 5.9 | 14.3 | 10 | 53.2 | 16 | 39 | 51.3 |
| Three-star PCTs | 5.6 | 14.4 | 9.8 | 53 | 17.3 | 39.4 | 51.4 |
| ONS Band 1 PCTs | 6.6 | 12.2 | 12.8 | 58.5 | 10.4 | 34.7 | 51.8 |
| ONS Band 2 | 5.8 | 14.7 | 10.2 | 52.7 | 15.7 | 38.7 | 51.5 |
| ONS Band 3 | 6.1 | 14.8 | 11.1 | 51.8 | 15.6 | 37.9 | 51.7 |
| ONS Band 4 | 5.7 | 13.9 | 10.4 | 53 | 16.5 | 39 | 51.1 |
| ONS Band 5 | 6.1 | 14.3 | 9.7 | 54 | 15 | 38.4 | 51.1 |
| ONS Band 6 | 5.5 | 13.9 | 9.6 | 53.1 | 16.9 | 39.8 | 51.2 |
| Specimen Band 3 PCT | 5.8 | 14 | 18.1 | 47.7 | 14.4 | 35.9 | 50.4 |
| PCT's percentile | 45th | 42nd | 98th | 5th | 25th | 10th | 8th |

Our case study (specimen) PCT stands out on several age variables. It has a large young adult population but much smaller older and younger populations. This profile will have implications for the mix of primary and community care teams if not the size.

Generally, elderly people are not only the most numerous but also the most dependent patients in community practitioners' caseloads. Indeed, studies showed that around three-quarters of community patients aged over 65 years were deemed highly dependent. These patients required almost four times more care than community patients in the lowest dependency category. However, these care ratios vary between areas (Craigmile et al. 1978; Piggott 1988; Durrand 1989).

Fieldwork in the author's study of elderly patients in four PCTs showed that:

- three-quarters required some care and 10% were severely disabled
- half were unable to perform basic activities of living and most were incontinent
- 25% were chair or bed bound
- three-quarters could not go out unaided
- one-fifth were aggressive and 10% were prone to injuring either themselves or others
- a surprisingly high proportion of elderly patients were demented or depressed
- co-morbidity was common.

Unmet need among people of any age is an issue for primary and community care staff, which caused Ledger (1987) to recommend a vulnerability index for community elderly patients to help practitioners prioritize their work. Fortunately, elderly patients are more likely to seek community services:

- Disabled: 3.6 times more likely
- Housebound: three times more likely
- Recently discharged from hospital, female and widowed patients are twice as likely to contact primary and community care practitioners (Victor and Vetter 1984), although these data are old and should be interpreted with caution.

These data, although old, may help practitioners predict higher demand in communities with above average numbers of elderly people. Williams et al.'s (1992) study underlined the levels of dependent community patients, with or without carers, needing community nurses' support. More recent data showed that, worryingly, the majority of community patients were not known to the local health services, especially when up to a third will fall or experience other problems (Lauder 1999; Vetter et al. 1992). Vetter et al.'s (1984) earlier data, although old, have important workforce planning and development messages. They showed that health visitors spend proportionally less time with elderly patients in the community. There seem to be missed opportunities because health visitors are the only professionals who visit patients without referral – important not only because of unmet needs but also because elderly people tend to report symptoms late and have difficulty travelling to general practices.

# Acute and chronic illness and disability (Tables 2.5 and 2.6)

Our case study PCT not only has a younger population but also a more chronically ill and disabled one, which also has staff-mix implications for both health and social services, e.g. younger, chronically ill community patients may be more capable of self-caring or have spouses and close relatives able to contribute to care. Similarly, Hudson and Hawthorne (1989) noted that 6–11% of community nurses' caseload is likely to feature disabled patients. Although dated, this study suggests that a community practitioner with rehabilitation skills might be an appropriate worker. Competent health-care assistants could also have an important role for this community patient group if community patient care is less technical.

Table 2.5 Acute and chronic illness

| PCT/Band | Acute illness (%) | GHQ ill-health (%) | Fair to bad health (%) | Poor health (%) |
|---|---|---|---|---|
| England | 15.1 | 16.8 | 23.8 | 8.9 |
| Three-star PCTs | 14.8 | 16.1 | 24.5 | 8.8 |
| ONS Band 1 PCTs | 18.6 | 22.1 | 27.8 | 8.6 |
| ONS Band 2 | 17.5 | 17.6 | 30.5 | 11.8 |
| ONS Band 3 | 14.3 | 16.3 | 27.2 | 10.1 |
| ONS Band 4 | 15.2 | 18.6 | 22.9 | 8.7 |
| ONS Band 5 | 14.3 | 17.5 | 19.2 | 6.9 |
| ONS Band 6 | 14.3 | 15.7 | 24.1 | 9.4 |
| Specimen Band 3 PCT | 14 | 16.3 | 26.1 | 11 |
| Specimen's percentile | 28th | 42nd | 65th | 85th |

GHQ, General Health Questionnaire.
Variables are defined in the PCT WP&D database.

**Table 2.6** Illness and disability

| PCT/Band | Young chronic ill (%) | Chronic illness (%) | Permanently sick (%) | Disabled (%) |
|---|---|---|---|---|
| England | 13 | 17.9 | 4.8 | 6.2 |
| Three-star PCTs | 12.9 | 18.3 | 4.9 | 6.4 |
| ONS Band 1 PCTs | 12.5 | 15.6 | 5.1 | 5 |
| ONS Band 2 | 17.4 | 21.8 | 8.4 | 8.9 |
| ONS Band 3 | 14.3 | 18.6 | 6.1 | 6.8 |
| ONS Band 4 | 12.7 | 17.4 | 4.7 | 5.8 |
| ONS Band 5 | 10.2 | 14.6 | 3.2 | 4.4 |
| ONS Band 6 | 14.1 | 19 | 5.3 | 6.7 |
| Specimen Band 3 PCT | 16 | 20.1 | 7.1 | 9 |
| Specimen's percentile | 78th | 70th | 80th | 88th |

Variables are defined in the PCT WP&D database.

# Patients' homes (Table 2.7)

A larger proportion of our case study PCT's housing stock is not only the least valuable but also accessed by at least one flight of stairs (it is accepted that some would have lifts). Twelve houses in every 1000 do not have central heating or a bath – although small, it is a good deprivation indicator. From earlier demographic data we saw that it is a younger, chronically ill population who may be living in these conditions. Shepherd's (1992) study found high levels of need in areas with poor housing. One family in three had high ill-health risk scores – notably high levels of smoking.

A reasonable assumption is that, if the houses in our case study PCT are also poor stock, the community practitioner's working environment and

**Table 2.7** Patients' homes

| PCT/Band | Band A housing (%) | No central heating or bath (%) | First floor + accommodation (%) | Lone pensioner (%) |
|---|---|---|---|---|
| England | 20 | 0.09 | 7.8 | 14.4 |
| Three Star PCTs | 23 | 0.1 | 6.2 | 15.1 |
| ONS Band 1 PCTs | 2 | 0.61 | 44.9 | 11.6 |
| ONS Band 2 | 58 | 0.05 | 6.1 | 15.1 |
| ONS Band 3 | 42 | 0.13 | 9.2 | 14.8 |
| ONS Band 4 | 10 | 0.2 | 11.6 | 14.3 |
| ONS Band 5 | 7 | 0.07 | 8.7 | 13.4 |
| ONS Band 6 | 31 | 0.08 | 5.9 | 14.6 |
| Specimen Band 3 PCT | 68 | 0.12 | 11.5 | 14.1 |
| Specimen's percentile | 95th | 60th | 75th | 42nd |

the quality of care they can deliver may be affected. Indeed, 91% of the community nurses in the *Occupational Health Review* (Anonymous 1994) survey experienced difficulties lifting community patients as a result of poor access in the rooms in which patients lived. Worryingly, less than half of community practitioners had undergone lifting and moving patient education and training, which might increase the risk of injury not only to staff but also to patients.

## Care home issues

Table 2.4 showed that elderly care in our case study site is less of an issue compared with PCTs in the same ONS Band. Nevertheless, Barret and Hudson's (1997) London study showed that rising community workloads were caused by the shift of care (especially elderly) from secondary to primary and community care. A growing elderly and very elderly population, along with the acute and nursing home sectors' falling capacity to accommodate them, is having an increasing effect on community practitioners' work (Barret and Hudson 1997). The number of elderly care home placements varies in England, and recently one PCT studied by the author lost 653 residential and care home beds in one year. Moreover, the new Care Standards Commission's tougher accreditation system means that more care homes are likely to close. As a consequence, managers were recording increases in the number of practitioner visits to residential homes. Managers estimated that two whole-time equivalent (WTE) extra staff were needed in each PCT to meet the 'free care home nursing' initiative and other policy changes – a point corroborated by the Audit Commission (1999).

**Table 2.8** Home care and care homes

| PCT/Band | Lone pensioner (%) | Unpaid carers (%) | Home care (hours per capita) | Care home population (%) |
|---|---|---|---|---|
| England | 14.4 | 20 | 0.05 | 0.56 |
| Three-star PCTs | 15.1 | 19 | 0.05 | 0.66 |
| ONS Band 1 PCTs | 11.6 | 20 | 0.08 | 0.13 |
| ONS Band 2 | 15.1 | 24 | 0.06 | 0.59 |
| ONS Band 3 | 14.8 | 22 | 0.02 | 0.46 |
| ONS Band 4 | 14.3 | 20 | 0.05 | 0.7 |
| ONS Band 5 | 13.4 | 17 | 0.05 | 0.51 |
| ONS Band 6 | 14.6 | 21 | 0.06 | 0.62 |
| Specimen Band 3 PCT | 14.1 | 26 | 0.05 | 0.43 |
| Specimen's percentile | 42nd | 90th | 40th | 28th |

Malone and Mackenzie (2000) investigated the care home patient demands on primary and community practitioners. They noted the number of patients who change from residential to nursing home status and a steadily rising level of dependency among patients in care homes (Table 2.8). Tissue viability and incontinence were issues with which community practitioners were regularly called upon to help.

Our case study PCT has well-below-average Social Service home care hours and consequently a higher proportion of unpaid carers (which may reflect the younger, chronically sick and disabled population noted earlier). Possibly because of its smaller elderly population, the PCT has a well-below-average care home population.

Durrand (1989) noted that the pressures on elderly care services were so great in some care teams that community practitioners' time was rationed, which meant that a burden of care was left with elderly patients' relatives, somewhat against the government's intentions. Also, work by Nuffield Institute staff (Hurst 2003) on elderly inpatient dependency shows that inpatients in some PCTs are more dependent than the England average and consequently trusts' elderly care inpatient workloads were above average. This related finding is important for several reasons because:

- community workload implications emerge following early discharge
- schemes designed to reduce 'winter pressures' on hospital services, such as intensive home support and intermediate care, which affect community practitioners – these were not only raised by interviewees but also reinforced in the literature
- a broad range of professionals, working with inpatients, outpatients and community patients, is affected.

Elderly care in the community is one of several workforce planning and development issues that embrace joint health and Social Service care. The single assessment process was raised by service managers during fieldwork conducted by the author. However, the workforce planning implications are not fully understood although early evidence suggests that the burden of assessment and care is falling to community practitioners.

## Children and child care issues (Table 2.9)

The care of children is another large chunk of work for primary and community practitioners. Shepherd (1992) pointed out that information from comprehensive profiling enabled particular cohorts to be studied such as families with pre-school children. These data are valuable for workforce planning.

**Table 2.9** Children and child care

| PCT/Band | < 5 years (%) | 5–15 years (%) | Lone parent (%) | Child protection registrants (%) | Accidents (%) |
|---|---|---|---|---|---|
| England | 5.9 | 14.3 | 5.8 | 0.04 | 18.2 |
| Three-star PCTs | 5.6 | 14.4 | 5.7 | 0.05 | 18.8 |
| ONS Band 1 PCTs | 6.6 | 12.2 | 8.2 | 0.07 | 13 |
| ONS Band 2 | 5.8 | 14.7 | 7.4 | 0.05 | 19 |
| ONS Band 3 | 6.1 | 14.8 | 7.5 | 0.02 | 18.3 |
| ONS Band 4 | 5.7 | 13.9 | 6.1 | 0.05 | 17.7 |
| ONS Band 5 | 6.1 | 14.3 | 5 | 0.04 | 18.2 |
| ONS Band 6 | 5.5 | 13.9 | 5.5 | 0.06 | 17.2 |
| Specimen Band 3 PCT | 5.8 | 14 | 9.9 | 0.1 | 17.9 |
| PCT's percentile | 45th | 42nd | 98th | 100th | 60th |

It might be argued that PCTs with the fastest growing populations have proportionally more youngsters although migration is a factor. Our case study PCT is in the top 40% of PCTs that are children and teenager rich. The Audit Commission (1994) highlights the variables relevant to child health services:

* poor housing and environment
* ill-health
* parental anxiety and stress
* unemployment and low income
* teenage mothers
* families lacking social support.

These variables lead to children's physical, emotional, mental and social under-development. They also have wide-ranging implications including cultural, educational, staff recruitment and retention. Similarly, Crofts et al. (2000) placed child protection high on the list of health visiting priorities. First-time mothers in the postnatal period (50% of contacts in Crofts et al.'s study) were thought to be mental illness prone, and therefore deserved more than routine visits. Similarly, Cox et al. (1991) noted that 1% of children on the child protection register are 5 years or younger and 30–40% of the mothers were severely depressed. They concluded that children's development would be affected under these circumstances – untoward outcomes that would be worse without health visitors' support.

The incidence of looked-after children and related problems, on the other hand, is falling (Audit Commission 1994). Nevertheless, our case study PCT is outstanding regarding child care and child protection issues – with major implications for health visitors and school nurses. Moreover, childhood accidents are an important public health problem especially in socioeconomically disadvantaged areas. Accidents are the most common cause of death in children under 1 year and result in considerable morbidity – reaching 640 000 A&E attendances per annum. Moreover, 10% of these children will be admitted to hospital (Kendrick et al. 1995). These data may explain why health visitors tend to prioritize children from disadvantaged areas because they are most at risk from injury and death. If practitioners are aware of high-risk families then they can intervene appropriately (Kendrick et al. 1995). Children on protection registers can be looked after in different settings (Hyde 2001):

- Local authority children's accommodation
- Supported accommodation
- Trustee care homes
- Support-at-home care.

The Audit Commission (1994) reminds us that individuals aged 18 years and under make up a quarter of the population although until recently they had no formal voice in matters concerning well-being. The 1989 Children's Act consolidated child legislation and balanced the relationship between families and the state. The Act also formalized health service and Social Service responsibilities and encouraged joint working. The main point is that child health care can still be duplicated by different agencies and is, therefore, wasteful (Audit Commission 1994). Although data are old, the distribution of child health and social care expenditure is interesting (ranked from high to low expenditure):

- Social work child support
- Residential care
- Fostering
- Day care
- Vaccination and immunization
- Development assessments
- Other professional advice and support
- Family centres
- Child health surveillance.

It seems that most child welfare expenditure is predominantly social-care related (Audit Commission 1994). Nevertheless, the Audit Commission's study showed that 3% of children are born injured or with a disability that may be beyond the scope of social services. Assessment of the needs of these children and their families by health-care professionals targets the needy, prioritizes services and redistributes resources.

# Morbidity and mortality data (see Tables 2.5 and 2.6)

These data help community and primary care workforce planners in many ways, e.g. the proportion of the population with General Health Questionnaire (GHQ) scores > 4 (indicating morbidity) in the ONS database ranges from 11% to 24%, and the proportion of people claiming disability allowance fluctuates between 3% and 13%. Managers interviewed by the author consistently underlined the effects of these data on community workload.

Our case study PCT has chronic illness levels likely to add to primary and community practitioners' workload, e.g. the specimen PCT remains in the undesirable half of the league table in most of the chronic illness and disability variables. Probably as a consequence of these chronic illness levels, more people in the specimen PCT claim disability allowances than both the England and ONS Band average. The PCT staff face a greater proportion of disabled people and it is reasonable to assume that these outcomes adversely affect primary and community workload as well as influencing important decisions about staff mix.

# Lifestyle and related issues (Table 2.10)

These variables have dependency and workload implications not only for community practitioners but also for health promotion which influences staff mix such as public health nursing work.

Table 2.10 Lifestyle and related issues

| PCT/Band | Smokers (daily cigarettes) | 4-week smoke quitters | Wheezers (%) | BMI > 30 (%) | Alcohol > 35 units (%) |
|---|---|---|---|---|---|
| England | 4 | 2[a] | 34 | 17 | 4.2 |
| Three-star PCTs | 3.6 | 2 | 35 | 17.9 | 4.2 |
| ONS Band 1 PCTs | 4.7 | 2 | 38 | 14.2 | 5.6 |
| ONS Band 2 | 5 | 2 | 35 | 17.8 | 5.2 |
| ONS Band 3 | 4.1 | 2 | 33 | 17.8 | 5.1 |
| ONS Band 4 | 3.9 | 2 | 36 | 15.8 | 3.5 |
| ONS Band 5 | 3.6 | 2 | 32 | 15.6 | 4.1 |
| ONS Band 6 | 3.7 | 2 | 33 | 18.1 | 3.9 |
| Specimen Band 3 PCT | 4 | 2 | 30 | 17.8 | 5.5 |
| Specimen's percentile | 50th | | 20th | 60th | 85th |

[a] 2, achieved.

There is a lower proportion of smokers and wheezers in our case study PCT. Judging from the data pattern, it would seem that pollution is important because the relationship to smoking and wheezing is not clear from the database. The 4-week smoking quitter figure indicates the degree to which PCT staff met or exceeded their targets. Unfortunately, this classification replaced a percentage figure used in previous years, which was more discriminatory. Obesity varies greatly between ONS Bands and our case study PCT has a higher proportion of overweight people to the extent that the PCT average is outside the confidence interval range.

Alcohol intake beyond the recommended level is also well above average in our case study PCT, which may explain its higher rate of accidents requiring hospital treatment. Several public health issues emerge from these data causing workforce planners to examine the size and mix of their primary and community-care teams. Carlisle (2003) is concerned that poor health indicators such as obesity, smoking and sexually transmitted diseases are rising among teenagers. Earlier we saw that the case study site had a younger population, which has even more implications for health promotion and disease prevention.

# Life expectancy and death rates (Table 2.11)

As we saw earlier, more people are obese in our case study site compared with the England and respective ONS Band averages. However, life expectancy data are mixed. The coronary heart disease (CHD) death rates are worse but cancer deaths are improving (even though the Healthcare Commission ratings do not discriminate too well). These better outcomes may reflect the PCT's average smoking data. Managers interviewed by the author said that

Table 2.11  Life expectancy and death rate

| PCT/Band | Male (years) | Female (years) | CHD deaths per 100 000 | Circulation deaths (% improvement) | Cancer deaths (improvement) |
|---|---|---|---|---|---|
| England | 75.5 | 80.2 | 118 | +3.3 | 3[a] |
| Three-star PCTs | 75 | 80.2 | 124 | +3.3 | 3 |
| ONS Band 1 PCTs | 74.6 | 80.7 | 125 | +4.5 | 3 |
| ONS Band 2 | 73.6 | 78.8 | 150 | +4.8 | 3 |
| ONS Band 3 | 74.3 | 79.6 | 129 | +6.6 | 3 |
| ONS Band 4 | 75.7 | 80.7 | 110 | +2.3 | 3 |
| ONS Band 5 | 76.5 | 80.9 | 104 | +2.4 | 3 |
| ONS Band 6 | 75.6 | 80.2 | 119 | +0.9 | 3 |
| Specimen Band 3 PCT | 74.7 | 80 | 124 | +0.7 | 3 |
| Specimen's percentile | 31st | 38th | 60th | 35th | NA |

[a] 5 = highest score.

more staff would allow them to educate the public (and professionals) about minimizing health (and social) care problems intimated in the tables. Indeed, many said that preventive roles were not only increasing but also proving a challenge. Some were disappointed that services designed to meet these new demands could not be established because of a lack of resources.

# Socioeconomic and quality-of-life data

Socioeconomic data augment local demographic, morbidity and mortality data immeasurably. These data are summarized in Table 2.12.

**Table 2.12** Socioeconomic and quality-of-life data

| PCT/Band | Deprivation (average rank) | Crime per 1000 | Unemployed (%) | Households without a car (%) | Without educational qualifications (%) |
|---|---|---|---|---|---|
| England | | 44 | 3 | 24 | 29 |
| Three-star PCTs | 166 | 40 | 3 | 22 | 28 |
| ONS Band 1 PCTs | 26 | 102 | 5.7 | 54 | 22 |
| ONS Band 2 | 42 | 55 | 4.1 | 33 | 35 |
| ONS Band 3 | 92 | 72 | 3.8 | 32 | 32 |
| ONS Band 4 | 133 | 39 | 3.1 | 25 | 27 |
| ONS Band 5 | 268 | 33 | 2.3 | 18 | 24 |
| ONS Band 6 | 143 | 39 | 3 | 22 | 31 |
| Specimen Band 3 PCT | 12 | 130 | 5.3 | 45 | 34 |
| Specimen's percentile | 5th | 98th | 95th | 95th | 72nd |

These data provide different insights into primary and community dependency and workload and staffing recommendations. The deprivation ranks, for example, give a robust indication of need. Our case study PCT is one of the most deprived localities in England and, because good health has is roots in several socioeconomic variables (Carlisle 2003), these data are vital. Poverty is an accepted determinant of poor health and poor people suffer more chronic illness and die earlier than richer people. Unfortunately, poverty seems to go hand in hand with inequality in that lower socioeconomic classes suffer unequal opportunity and access to health services – the so-called inverse care law, which suggests that those who most need health services receive the least (Tudor-Hart 1971). Often there is an unequal distribution of health care, which means that community and primary staff fail to meet extra needs among people in deprived communities (Hyde 2001).

However, Deal (1994) explained that factors affecting community demands are increasingly better understood, which should help to reverse inequitable situations.

Rowe et al. (1995) explained that families in deprived areas need more attention from health visitors. She prioritized families using an assessment that included:

- child protection registrants
- mentally and physically disabled children
- chronically ill children such as asthma sufferers
- social problem families
- families with marital problems
- unsupported single parents
- substance abusers.

Inequitable workloads have been a major concern among managers (Kemp 1969; Shepherd 1992). In one area 6% of the health visitors' caseloads included families that met one or more of the criteria above. However, only some of the health visitors working in poorer areas with families meeting these criteria had smaller caseloads, which implies that health visiting time and resources were rationed or inequitably managed. Moreover, all had families with a greater risk of ill-health compared with the caseloads of health visitors working in affluent areas. The distribution of health visiting resources was unrelated to deprivation and, when other variables such as ethnicity were considered, community patient demand and practitioner workload became even more unequally distributed (Shepherd 1992). Encouragingly, on the other hand, recent data showed that health visitors working in deprived areas had smaller caseloads – an important equity issue that affects both the supply and demand side of workforce planning (Cotton et al. 2000; Crofts et al. 2000).

Crime data are featuring more in profiling and workforce planning as well as developing policies such as Sure Start (Roberts and Anstead 1996; Hyde 2001). They are included here because crime rates affect not only the population's quality of life but also community staff working conditions. The latter is an issue that is likely to become more acute as a predominantly female workforce extends its out of hours' work in the community, which has considerable job safety implications.

The educational qualifications also might seem an odd variable to include in a workforce planning and development book. However, there appears to be stronger connection with deprivation, unemployment, and scholastic achievement and educational qualifications, which is bound to influence NHS and Social Service recruitment.

# Deprivation and demand (Table 2.13)

Census data include valuable health-care demand variables and an important use of these data is community workload estimation. Local authorities and their co-terminus health PCTs are ranked from most to least deprived (Hyde 2001). If the number of finished consultant episodes (FCEs), as a measure of need, is correlated to deprivation then the correlation is significant ($r = 0.55$, $p < 0.05$). The Audit Commission's (1992b) study showed that primary and secondary care spending are connected so it is likely that FCEs influence primary and community care activity.

**Table 2.13** Deprivation and demand

| PCT/Band | Deprivation (average rank) | FCE per capita |
|---|---|---|
| England | | 1 FCE to 4.5 people |
| Three-star PCTs | 166 | 4.5 |
| ONS Band 1 PCTs | 26 | 5.7 |
| ONS Band 2 | 42 | 3.7 |
| ONS Band 3 | 92 | 4.4 |
| ONS Band 4 | 133 | 4.7 |
| ONS Band 5 | 268 | 5.5 |
| ONS Band 6 | 143 | 4.3 |
| Specimen Band 3 PCT | 12 | 4.3 |
| Specimen's percentile | 5th | 40th |

FCE, finished consultant episode.

As raised earlier, it is accepted that health inequalities are closely related to social and economic factors (Kendall and Lissauer 2003). One Department of Health target is to reduce health inequalities as measured by infant mortality rates and life expectancy by 10% (Carlisle 2003). Workforce planners therefore need to account for inequalities and prioritize caseloads in some way by tailoring services to deprived areas (Goodwin 1994; DoH 2001b). Community practitioners, notably health visitors, work closely with deprived populations by trying to address the needs of vulnerable groups while at the same time providing a universal service to all families with children aged under 5 (Almond 2002; DoH 2002b). However, Reading and Allen's (1997) study showed an irrational relationship between social class and health visiting activity, for example, and, encouragingly, deprived families received 30% more health visiting time although preventive health programmes were directed at affluent families, whereas parent-class sessions were taken up by families in the middle-affluence range. There was no clear evidence of strategic interventions for families in need. Kendall and Lissauer (2003) suggest that the medical model's dominance in health needs assessment and workforce planning may explain unequal access.

## The FCE rates and delayed discharges

Shorter inpatient stays and rapid throughput mean that moderately dependent patients of all ages are discharged earlier into the care of primary and community staff, which has considerable implications for primary and community workload. Indeed, average inpatient stay fell by 3.3 days over 10 years between 1985 and 1995, whereas the number of surgical procedures doubled (Audit Commission 1992b; Frame and O'Donnell 1996). The number of FCEs rose by 38% over the 5 years to 1998, whereas the ratio of nurses to FCEs fell in the same period (Buchan and Edwards 2000).

Table 2.14 FCE rates and delayed discharges

| PCT/Band | FCE per capita | Non-delayed hospital transfer (band) |
|---|---|---|
| England | 1 FCE to 4.5 people | 3[a] |
| Three-star PCTs | 4.5 | 3 |
| ONS Band 1 PCTs | 5.7 | 3 |
| ONS Band 2 | 3.7 | 3 |
| ONS Band 3 | 4.4 | 3 |
| ONS Band 4 | 4.7 | 3 |
| ONS Band 5 | 5.5 | 3 |
| ONS Band 6 | 4.3 | 2 |
| Specimen Band 3 PCT | 4.3 | 3 |
| Specimen's percentile | 40th | 50th |

[a]5 = best score.
FCE, finished consultant episode.

Roughly one in four members in our case study PCT population experienced an FCE. Although a secondary care workload indicator, FCEs have implications for primary and community care because patients are referred to and received from secondary care services. Not only is the specimen PCT 'busier' but it also experiences an average hospital discharge rate. Problems may include the lack of care home places and home support noted earlier – both well below average levels in our case study PCT.

Not only are more hospital patients discharged into the community but also advancing medical technology and shifting boundaries between secondary and primary care mean that community practitioners increasingly care for highly dependent patients in their homes (DoH 1993a, 2002b; Jenkins-Clarke 1997). Edwardson and Nardone (1990) showed a strong correlation between patient dependency and the number of practitioner visits ($r_p$ = 0.15, $n$ = 450, $p$ < 0.05). They argued that, as the variety and complexity of patients seen at home change, it becomes increasingly important to specify the care needs of patients in a dependency group and the services provided for them.

Local managers, during interviews, commented on the number of complex care cases handled by community practitioners. Consequently, practitioners are specializing in order to meet community patients' needs. In one community study (Dewis 2001) the ratio of patients with multiple nursing needs to single care need patients averaged 1:8 (SD = 3), a figure that was rising. The Audit Commission (1999) neatly summarized the reasons behind an increasing and unpredictable community patient dependency and workload and the importance of health needs analysis and related data:

- open referral system
- shortening hospital stays
- fourfold difference in the referral rates between different localities:
  - $n$ = 40 trusts
  - mean = 37.4 referrals per 1000 population
  - SD = 12.6
- inappropriate referrals
- up to one in twelve terminally ill patients in a community.

## Conclusion

Community patient dependency and workload are important components of PCT workforce planning and development (WP&D). However, they have different meanings than the same phrases applied to inpatient workforce planning. In the community, dependency and workload assessments are usually drawn from the locality's socioeconomic and morbidity data rather than patient acuities, although (somewhat dated) methods for generating the latter exist in the literature.

Collection of patient dependency and workload-related data is not popular among community practitioners – issues about which PCT managers need to be sensitive. Nevertheless, these data are important not least because the community is never 'full' and primary and community care workload fluctuations have equity implications for staff and patients. Fortunately, in recent years, centrally held primary and community care databases are growing in variety and content, which has significant value for assessing demand and workload.

The choice of patient dependency and workload measures in the literature (see Annotated bibliography, page 167) range from simple activity-
of-living-based methods to complex health needs assessment or community
profiles. Each has strengths and weaknesses and an important feature is how
methods relate to specific patient groups such as elderly people or patients
living in deprived areas. Some dependency and workload measures are better at accounting for community patients' or carers' contributions, whereas
others give strong indications about a professional group's responsibilities
(such as health visitors). In short, there are horses for courses. The main
problem, however, is that these approaches are redundant in patient-
focused, integrated, competency-based primary care workforce planning and
development.

Nevertheless, managers and practitioners need information to help them
prioritize and direct staff. Deprivation data, useful information for PCT managers, feature strongly in the community profile method not only because of
the inverse care law but also because of staffing implications. Analysis of
PCT-related morbidity, mortality and socioeconomic data therefore generates considerable insights into community patient wants and needs. Despite
their limitations and the way these community data are treated as proxy
measures, they reveal remarkable differences between ONS Bands and PCTs
in the same band. This important finding clearly shows that generic one-size-
fits-all workforce planning algorithms would not only be inaccurate but also
grossly unfair.

More than 90 demographic, morbidity, mortality, quality-of-life, staff and
performance variables and corresponding data from Department of Health
and ONS databases are included in a PCT WP&D database. In recent years,
these data have not only become easier to extract but also to interrogate for
primary and community care WP&D purposes. However, although the
demographic and socioeconomic data are well understood by PCT managers, they are rarely fully exploited. This book tries to set the record straight
and help managers interpret their PCT's profile.

Workforce-related data in the Department of Health and ONS databases
have been aligned to their respective PCTs and summarized for benchmarking purposes. A wide range has been aggregated into the PCT WP&D
database and made as flexible as possible. To highlight this feature, as we saw
earlier, one PCT is profiled as a specimen case-study trust and compared not
only with English averages but also with its ONS socioeconomically similar
counterparts. The specimen PCT is also compared with three-star trusts,
which for the purpose of the study are deemed 'best practice'. Indeed, the
tables throughout the book show that three-star PCTs achieve their high performance ratings efficiently and effectively. However, readers will also notice
the three-star low dependency and workload indicators. Nevertheless, it is
hoped that the case study PCT and its benchmarked positions, used as a

thread throughout the remainder of this book, will help the reader to think and act on similar data relevant to his or her trust.

Managers and practitioners can use the PCT WP&D database not only to evaluate traditional PCT's workforce but more importantly also to address health policy developments, e.g. the levels of chronic illness and disability in some PCTs are double the national average, which has implications for *Liberating the Talents'* (DoH 2002c) core functions. Unusual variables, such as person and property crime rates, are also included in the PCT WP&D database for their staff health and safety implications, notably for out-of-hours services.

# CHAPTER THREE

# Community staff activity

## Introduction and background

Bryar (1994) and later Craig and Smith (1998) succinctly listed primary and community health-care professionals' main roles:

- Promoting and maintaining health, and preventing disease
- Involving individuals, their families and communities in professional decision-making and self-care
- Reducing inequalities in health care for the under-served
- Multidisciplinary and multisectorial collaboration.

Data covering many of these are available to the reader from www.health-careworkforce.org.uk, some of which has been discussed in Chapters 1 and 2. Data about the ways community practitioners spend their time are vital not only for workforce planning and development but also for improving efficiency and effectiveness. However, recording activity and analysing data meaningfully are a challenge for practitioners and primary care trust (PCT) managers (Department of Health or DoH 1993b; Goodman 1996). According to Naish and Kline (1990) ideal workforce planning and development data include:

- a combination of hard, quantitative (such as epidemiological) and soft, qualitative (such as patient feedback) data
- practitioner workload
- community profiles
- time out and job satisfaction
- vacancies
- staff-mix information.

The first three have already been discussed and are developed in this chapter. The remaining three are explored in detail in later chapters.

Fortunately, data implied in this list are readily available from centrally held databases. Unfortunately, however, managers and practitioners are no longer required to gather certain Korner activity data, although it is hoped they will continue collecting information for monitoring purposes (Andrews 2004). Qualitative data about the workforce, on the other hand, will have to be gathered individually by PCT workforce planners or culled from the literature (see Annotated bibliography, page 167), e.g. information gathered during PCT manager interviews generated important insights in this study, which are raised periodically in the book.

Recently introduced policies such as *Liberating the Talents* (DoH 2002c), Personal Medical Service (PMS) and the new General Medical Service (GMS) policies (DoH 2002b; Lewis and Rosen 2003) are causing a radical change to strategic and operational workforce planning, e.g. *Liberating the Talents* reclassified the work of community practitioners into three new categories:

1. First contact: acute assessment, diagnosis, treatment, care and referral.
2. Continuing care: National Service Framework (NSF)-oriented rehabilitation and chronic disease management.
3. Public health: promotion and protection aimed at improving health and reducing inequalities.

These new policies and the roles that emerge are designed to do the following:

- Make health care more efficient and effective by deploying staff differently. Overcoming 'the sea of faces' problem that besets the NHS could be achieved if individual roles are broadened and deepened along new policy lines.
- Alleviate primary care workforce supply-side problems such as the shortage of GPs.
- Give community nurses opportunities to develop their knowledge and skills while improving job satisfaction, recruitment and retention.
- Encourage multidisciplinary working and mutual problem-solving rather than 'buck passing' and isolated working.

However, one potential downside of new workforce planning and development policies is the negative perceptions held by some practitioners, which could make change uncertain. Also, professional tribalism and protected budgets may jeopardize these new roles as boundaries between staff groups remain firm (Hyde 2001; DoH 2003; Howkins and Thornton 2003).

## First contact

First contact or direct care access usually initiates the preliminary assessment and then follow-up care (Bryar 1994). This is an important workload category because 90% of all patient journeys begin (and end) in primary care and community practitioners are central to this work (DoH 2002c). The increasing number of minor illness self-referrals to GPs strains resources while demand for same-day care is growing. But not all patients, especially those with self-limiting diseases, need to see a GP, thereby releasing medical staff to see patients with special needs. In short, primary and community care practitioners can improve efficiency and effectiveness by collaborating (Ross 1980a, 1980b).

As with GPs, practice nurses are another member of the main first contact staff group. Their work is varied and potentially satisfying, which positively influences recruitment and retention (Hyde 2001; Buckle and Gallen 2003):

- Screening, disease prevention and health promotion
- Dedicated follow-up clinics
- Treatment room work including minor surgery
- Home visits
- Counselling.

Atkin et al. (1994) explored practice nurse work in detail. Their respondents undertook the duties shown in Table 3.1.

**Table 3.1** Practice nurse work

| Work | Respondent (%) |
| --- | --- |
| Immunization and vaccination | 96 |
| Health promotion | 91 |
| Venepuncture | 86 |
| New patient assessment | 86 |
| Auroscopy | 83 |
| Peak-flow testing | 83 |
| Preparing equipment for GPs | 78 |
| Minor surgery assistance | 74 |
| Breast examination | 67 |
| Chronic disease management | 66–52 (depending on the disease) |
| Electrocardiography | 60 |
| Minor surgery | 53 |
| Mental illness detection | 43 |
| Family planning | 27 |
| Antenatal and postnatal | 23 |
| Stethoscopic examination | 9 |
| Ophthalmoscopy | 8 |

Prescribing is not mentioned because the nurse prescribing policy emerged after the survey of Atkins et al. Nevertheless, the activities in Table 3.1 have varying degrees of responsibility that range from assistant to autonomous practitioner (Hirst et al. 1998). Jeffreys et al.'s (1995) study, although 8 years old, probably still reflects practice nurse activities (Table 3.2).

**Table 3.2** Practice nurse activities from study by Jeffreys et al. (1995)

| Intervention | Range |
| --- | --- |
| Procedures per hour | 2.7–3.2 |
| Consultations per hour | 2.3–2.9 |
| Mean consultation time (min) | 21–26 |
| Mean time per procedure (min) | 19–22 |
| Annual consultation rate | 0.8 per patient |
| Traditional tasks (%) | 59–63 |
| Extended roles (%) | 24–28 |
| Diagnostic and management work (%) | 9–9.5 |
| Inappropriate referrals (%) | 30 |

Personal Medical Service evaluations showed that practice nurses and nurse practitioners undertake the full diagnostic, treatment and review process among patients with undifferentiated diagnosis. However, GPs 'cherry picked' cases and referred less interesting patients to nurses, thereby generating unfair access. Other problems were the barriers to extending nurse practitioners' roles such as signing sickness certificates, certain prescriptions and inappropriate referrals as a result of poor communication (Martin 1987; Wiles and Robinson 1994; Walsh et al. 2003). Doubts about practice nurses' abilities to extend their role seem unfounded, e.g. Walsh et al. (2003) showed that practice nurses lacked confidence rather than knowledge and skills whereas Long et al. (2002) underlined the value that other professionals place on patient assessments by practice nurses.

Developments such as the PMS, the new GMS contract, GPs with special interests (GPSIs), community hospital inpatient and professional executive committee (PEC) work make it inevitable that practice nurses take on more first contact work, especially in single medical practitioner general practices (Hirst et al. 1998). Indeed, Martin (1987), Hyde (2001) and Latimer and Ashburner (1997) noted that practice nurses were taking on more time-consuming roles previously done by GPs. Practice nurses are more qualified to undertake some of their medical colleagues' work because the former can competently deal with a range of social care as well as medical and nursing issues.

Practice nurses are flexible workers who deliver high-quality services although, because of the issues raised above, there is a danger that they are seen as physicians' assistants. As Table 3.3 shows, practice nurse staffing is generous in the case study site, where they are well placed to take on GP duties because the latter are less numerous per head of population.

**Table 3.3** Primary care practitioners per head of population

| PCT/Band | GPs per capita | Practice nurses per capita |
|---|---|---|
| England | 1:2009 | 1:4582 |
| Three-star PCTs | 1932 | 4509 |
| ONS Band 1 PCTs | 2136 | 4889 |
| ONS Band 2 | 1981 | 4467 |
| ONS Band 3 | 2015 | 4375 |
| ONS Band 4 | 2040 | 4845 |
| ONS Band 5 | 1968 | 4797 |
| ONS Band 6 | 1954 | 4437 |
| Specimen Band 3 PCT | 2033 | 3556 |
| PCT's percentile | 65th | 6th |

The generous practice nurse staffing in some, especially three-star PCTs, means that managers are well placed to re-configure primary care work so that practice nurses are geared for first contact work.

## Access to primary care practitioners

General and nurse practitioner mix is important for two Healthcare Commission (formerly the Commission for Health Improvement or CHI) standards. By September 2002, 81% of GPs were meeting the 2-day appointment and 69% had met the 1-day appointment standard; 90% of GPs were expected to meet the 2-day standard by April 2003 (Clews 2003). Indeed, as Table 3.4 indicates, all PCTs met the access targets. Elsewhere, some primary

**Table 3.4** Access to primary care practitioners

| PCT/Band | GP 48-h access (band) | Primary care 24-h access (band) |
|---|---|---|
| England | 2a | 2[a] |
| Three-star PCTs | 2 | 2 |
| ONS Band 1 PCTs | 2 | 2 |
| ONS Band 2 | 2 | 2 |
| ONS Band 3 | 2 | 2 |
| ONS Band 4 | 2 | 2 |
| ONS Band 5 | 2 | 2 |
| ONS Band 6 | 2 | 2 |
| Specimen Band 3 PCT | 2 | 2 |
| PCT's percentile | NA | NA |

[a] 2 = achieved.

and community care waiting times are lengthening which are linked to staff shortages and inappropriate staff mix.

Managers are never happy about waiting lists and waiting times, and spend considerable time prioritizing their services and finding ways of doing things differently. Nevertheless, waiting lists are part and parcel of health and social services. Trust managers interviewed in the present study felt that working life was a balance between maintaining standards during a limited practitioner–patient contact time and extending practitioners beyond a reasonable call of duty, e.g. it was not uncommon for practitioners in the author's study to complete their administrative and clerical work in their off-duty time. In other interviews managers said that waiting lists were lengthening as a result of staffing shortages and rising demand. Sexual health service staff, for example, were victims of their own success. They were struggling to meet their service standard of same-day appointment as demand rose after drop-in clinics were introduced. However, patient satisfaction was high.

Lengthening waiting lists and waiting times show that either services are understaffed or practitioners are working inappropriately. First contact need not be face to face or mean more work, because recent service changes such as NHS Direct, practice-based telephone triage and walk-in centres are likely to influence referral patterns and improve efficiency and effectiveness. However, recent literature turns away from demand and supply reasons for lengthening waiting lists and looks towards working practices (the workforce development side). For example, one PCT's central booking service for general and specialist community services, which included call screening by a health-care professional, greatly improved efficiency and effectiveness (Jenkins-Clarke and Carr-Hill 2001; Kendall and Lissauer 2003; Patterson 2003).

It is not clear whether these new ways of working are increasing or decreasing referrals, but practitioners felt that these developments challenged professional boundaries. Opinions of these services in the interviews and in the literature were mixed. Some saw them as exciting developments whereas others viewed them as a threat to professional groups. Also, new services were siphoning staff away from traditional services (discussed in Chapter 7). The literature indicates, however, that patients were more satisfied with services designed to improve access and convenience. The effect of NHS Direct and walk-in centres on acute services, let alone primary and community care activities, is not fully understood and at times findings are contradictory, e.g. the expected impact of these new services in one PCT area took an unexpected turn, i.e. users, against expectations, did not seek treatment or advice outside working hours (a common complaint from patients attending health-care services during office hours). The implications for general practice, therefore, are uncertain.

## Chronic disease management and continuing care

Primary and community care are traditionally associated with supporting ill and disabled people within the context of patients' work and family lives. Prevention and longer-term care, rather than technical medical interventions, dominate these services. Consequently, the second *Liberating the Talents* category, chronic disease management and continuing care (CDM), is likely to influence community staff activity (Bryar 1994).

Goodman's (1996) systematic review of the literature and Hesketh's (2002) empirical study described the antecedents to CDM, e.g. the population is ageing while co-morbidity is increasing. Technological care, now possible in the community, means that more sophisticated procedures among increasingly dependent community patients are possible. Well-informed district nurses, with their strong, central roles have the closest contact with these community patients (Naish and Kline 1990; Hyde 2001) and one implication is that they can increase their autonomy by leading CDM (Latimer and Ashburner 1997). Moreover, district nurses are taking on more CDM as a result of falling numbers of GPs, PMS and intermediate care initiatives. In the case of PMS, a broad range of work such as services for patients with poor access to health care is emerging (Hyde 2001; Walsh et al. 2003).

The relationship between primary and community care staff influences CDM workloads (Bryar 1997; DoH 1993a), e.g. the number of practice nurses has trebled in the last 10 years, which has dramatically reduced the time district nurses spend in the treatment room (Wiles and Robinson 1994; Jenkins-Clarke and Carr-Hill 2001). How PMS, modernization programmes and the new GMS affect these working styles is not clear but the number of practice nurses is not expected to fall. Unfortunately, data that explain the primary and community care interface are not held centrally and only a few primary care variables that generated insights into community workload were located during the present study. These are summarized by PCT in the workforce planning and development (WP&D) database.

The division between health and social care has become an issue in recent years because the line between health and social care cannot easily be drawn. As raised earlier, community patients oscillate between health and social carers, so agreeing objectives between different agencies is crucial (DoH 1993b). Earl-Slater (1995) described a new referral and rapid response community service designed to minimize unnecessary hospital stay. This strengthened multidisciplinary teams and reduced the cost of secondary care but increased community care workload and costs. The outcome for the NHS, however, was an overall saving.

## Referrals to community practitioners

Two and three-quarter million patients get home care from community nurses at a cost of £650m a year (Kneafsey et al. 2003). In practice, 80% of this work is task-oriented, continuing care (Audit Commission 1999). Of all primary care team members, district nurses make and receive the most referrals. Fifteen years ago GPs referred 69% of the patients in district nurses' caseloads (Moran-Ellis et al. 1985), but today GPs refer about 40%, accounting for a tenth of the district nurse and a fifth of the practice nurse workload. GPs, on the other hand, refer fewer patients to health visitors, which may explain why collaboration is stronger among GPs, district nurses and practice nurses (Cartlidge et al. 1987a, 1987b; Jenkins-Clarke and Carr-Hill 1996).

Recent data show shifting referral patterns with a disturbing amount of inappropriate referrals to district nurses (Audit Commission 1999) (Table 3.5).

Table 3.5 Referral patterns

| Referral sources | Percentage | Inappropriate referral (%) |
|---|---|---|
| GP | 40 | 17 |
| Hospital | 14 | 25 |
| Self/carer | 13 | 30 |
| Other | 9 | |
| Liaison nurse | 5 | 24 |
| Other district nurse | 4 | 22 |
| Practice nurse | 3 | 19 |
| Social Services | 2 | 14 |

Inappropriate referrals fell into three categories (Audit Commission 1999):

1. Patient referred to the wrong person.
2. Patient discharged inappropriately.
3. Community nursing care was not required.

Although these data have been challenged, the issues raised are important. The Audit Commission (1992a, 1999) estimated that inappropriate referrals amount to the equivalent of one whole-time equivalent (WTE) G grade nurse in each trust and that a 1% reduction in the amount of inappropriate work releases an extra 2.5 WTE community nurses. Ross (1980a, 1908b) felt that some of these referrals are simply dumping of unpopular patients or undesirable problems by GPs. Nurses have the prerogative to refuse referred patients if they feel that they are beyond their competence or scope. However, most 'dumped' patients are unlikely to fall into this category.

Each year elderly patients are likely to consult their GPs about three times and the practice nurse twice. At around 16% of the population, elderly people account for 20% of a GP's consultations (Cochrane et al. 2002). This may explain why the bulk of referrals to primary and community nurses are elderly care. Earlier studies showed that 75% of district nurses' time was spent caring for elderly people (Durrand 1989). Referrals and probably time spent with elderly people will continue to grow, not least because of their rising numbers and recent health policies designed to maintain their independence in the community.

## District nursing activity

Goodman (1996) and Williams et al. (1992) concluded that district nurses can find it difficult to articulate what they do as a result of their complex and discrete clinical problem-solving and decision-making, which form part of their health and social care roles, e.g. a sixth of district nurses' patients have no specific condition, which suggests that supervision and pastoral care are strong features. Only 20% of the referrals to district nurses were for assessment whereas 80% were task-oriented activities of living-related care, and also some technical care such as wound checks (Hudson and Hawthorn 1989). These findings suggest that district nurses' time may be wasted and their knowledge and skills not fully used (Audit Commission 1999), which has job satisfaction implications. Nevertheless, this work, usually elderly care, is important if elderly patients' independence in the community is to be maintained (Audit Commission 1986; Durrand 1989).

However, despite inappropriate referrals and subsequent activity, district nurses' job descriptions are not only comprehensive but also include duties that are satisfying (Moran-Ellis et al. 1985; DoH 1993c, 1993d; Deal 1994; Lochead 1994; RCN 1997):

- Health needs assessment
- Screening and well woman clinics
- Diagnosis and treatment
- Travel health and immunization
- Health promotion, education and counselling
- Care management
- Risk assessor
- Referral agent
- Liaison officer
- Rehabilitation
- Palliation

- Team management
- Audit, research and development
- Basic and continuing education.

Obviously, these roles influence both the nature and the frequency of community practitioner interventions. As we saw in Chapter 2, the frequency and duration of contact between the community patient and professional also influence community practitioners' workloads (Durrand 1989). The efficiency and effectiveness of community and primary interventions are important and quite rightly occupy managers' minds because of the activity cost and quality implications. However, output and outcome data need careful examination before action is taken. Ten years ago full-time district nurses averaged 52 contacts per week, the same as the previous decade (Anonymous 1994). Visits lasted 15–43 minutes and, although times varied, differences between localities were not statistically significant (Rapport and Maggs 1997).

Recent data are confusing, however, because they show that activity is either increasing or decreasing depending on the source. One reason for falling contacts is shifting social care interventions to local authority carers, which has reduced the number of community practitioner contacts. Indeed, 36% of patients in Rapport and Maggs' (1997) study were looked after jointly with Social Service staff whereas Barret and Hudson (1997) showed that health-care professional home visits had fallen steadily since the mid-1990s although the visits lasted longer. Another reason for falling contacts is that the number of interventions by specialist community practitioners has doubled in recent years (Wiles and Robinson 1994) and may not be included in the Korner data. These changes may also explain why time spent by district nurses on patients' personal care in the author's fieldwork fell by 30% whereas technical care time such as medicating increased 6%, and educational and counselling activities showed a 13% increase to around 17% of nursing time (see below).

A constantly worrying issue is the amount of time district nurses spend administratively, which can occupy a quarter of their working day or around 10 hours per week in the case of full-time staff. Administrative time increases with seniority, something with which nurses become increasingly frustrated (Anonymous 1994; Rink et al. 1996). Consequently, Andrews (2004) studied the activities practitioners thought were a waste of time:

- Routine paperwork and administration
- Fruitless time spent contacting colleagues especially Social Services
- Chasing hospital information needed for planning community care
- Travelling and finding a car parking space
- No access visits
- Inappropriate referrals and 'dumping' of problem patients by colleagues.

These unproductive activities not only are disliked but also contribute to broader, negative job perceptions. Rapport and Maggs (1997) carried out qualitative interviews with district nurses, which showed wide-ranging views of nursing work. Themes emerging were the long hours and missed lunch breaks. Although staff offered patients as much time as possible, visits were rushed and 'make do'. Standards were felt to be slipping, which demoralized and de-motivated the workforce. Continuing professional development had fallen and teamwork was fragmenting. Worst of all, practitioners felt that their managers lacked awareness of community nursing and had unrealistic expectations.

The most frequently occurring activities (Table 3.6) have changed over time (Whitaker 1977; Moran-Ellis et al. 1985; Anonymous 1994; McDonald et al. 1997; Dewis 2001).

**Table 3.6** Most frequently occurring activities

| Activity (rank order) | 1977 | 1985 | 1992 | 2001 |
|---|---|---|---|---|
| Continence work | | | | 1 |
| General support | 1 | 1 | | |
| Admin/clerical | | 2 | 1 | |
| Travelling | | | 2 | |
| Bathing | | 2 | 3 | |
| Advice/support | 4 | 4 | 4 | |
| Wound care | 3 | 5 | | 2 |
| Medication | 5 | | | 3 |

However, data vary owing to inconsistencies in the way activities are labelled and recorded. A large data-set collected by the author summarized the most frequently occurring activities in five PCTs broken down by professional group. District nursing activities were the most consistent over time and practitioners seemed able to balance their caseload management/administration and technical/psychosocial care duties. Some district nurses favoured psychosocial interventions, or there could be different ways of categorizing direct patient care.

Goodman (1996) felt that district nurses were insular workers who did not take the opportunity to collaborate with colleagues. As raised earlier, their work can be professionally rather than patient determined, which led some patients to say that district nursing interventions were inappropriate. One driver that influences district nurses' work is the new care home regulations and the way tighter finances are forcing care homes to close. These developments increased the number of visits to elderly people, in one PCT studied by the author, by 20–40 per community team.

# Primary and community care of elderly people

Some PCTs have disproportionately more people in care homes, which is likely to affect community nursing work (Table 3.7). First, the effects of free nursing home care were just being felt at the time of the author's study. Second, more dependent elderly patients looked after in care homes ought to lessen the community practitioners' burden. Third, the extension of community services to 24-hour care, especially as out-of-hours and chronic disease management services grow, could also alter the nature and frequency of community nursing contacts with patients. Although the data are old, Hudson and Hawthorn (1989) calculated that each of the 87 district nurses in their study looked after six stroke patients. Later, Hesketh (2002) and Kneafsey et al. (2003) underlined the community nurses' specific rehabilitation role:

- Assessing the patient's abilities and needs
- Accessing services on the patient's behalf
- Referral
- Helping patient to adapt by teaching and supporting him or her
- Technical care.

Table 3.7 Care of elderly people

| PCT/Band | Lone pensioner (%) | Unpaid carers (%) | Home care (hours per capita) | Care home population (%) |
|---|---|---|---|---|
| England | 14.4 | 20 | 0.05 | 0.56 |
| Three-star PCTs | 15.1 | 19 | 0.05 | 0.66 |
| ONS Band 1 PCTs | 11.6 | 20 | 0.08 | 0.13 |
| ONS Band 2 | 15.1 | 24 | 0.06 | 0.59 |
| ONS Band 3 | 14.8 | 22 | 0.02 | 0.46 |
| ONS Band 4 | 14.3 | 20 | 0.05 | 0.7 |
| ONS Band 5 | 13.4 | 17 | 0.05 | 0.51 |
| ONS Band 6 | 14.6 | 21 | 0.06 | 0.62 |
| Specimen Band 3 PCT | 14.1 | 26 | 0.05 | 0.43 |
| Specimen's percentile | 42nd | 90th | 40th | 28th |

Cochrane et al. (2002) explored chronic disease management from other angles. In the case of stroke patients, the authors envisaged case management as:

- Admission avoidance and prevention
- Home safety and risk assessment
- Patient monitoring
- Rapid response and intensive home support.

However, Hesketh (2002) and Kneafsey et al. (2003) judged stroke care to be unfocused, limited by a lack of time or judged to be less important. There is a tendency for this care to be left to the family who had not been fully prepared. Leadership was lacking and practitioners rarely collaborated. As with other Future Healthcare Worker (FHCW) reports, a generic, multiskilled community worker would be the ideal practitioner, overcoming Latimer and Ashburner's (1997) fears of a steadily fragmenting primary and community care service.

## Travelling time

Although the number of community practitioner contacts is falling, McIntosh et al. (2000) reported a 33% increase in the number of patients seen at home. Data about PCTs' geographical density and travelling time are important for workforce planners, because practitioners spend up to 25% of their day time travelling between homes and clinics (Audit Commission 1992a). The amount of time spent travelling can vary threefold (Worral and Goldstone 1980); although these are old data they should prompt managers at least to benchmark this so-called associated work (Table 3.8).

**Table 3.8** Practitioner travelling time variables

| PCT | Population density | Households without cars (%) |
| --- | --- | --- |
| England | 2427 | 24 |
| Three-star PCTs | 2494 | 22 |
| ONS Band 1 PCTs | 11 247 | 54 |
| ONS Band 2 | 3980 | 33 |
| ONS Band 3 | 5987 | 32 |
| ONS Band 4 | 2687 | 26 |
| ONS Band 5 | 1828 | 18 |
| ONS Band 6 | 1224 | 22 |
| Specimen Band 3 PCT | 8892 | 45 |
| PCT's percentile | 85th | 95th |

Population density (people per PCT square mile) and car ownership influence not only staff travelling time but also patient access (Hyde 2001). There is an important link between travelling and costs (1997 prices), which varied widely from 33p to £2.04 per contact (Clinical Benchmarking Company or CBC 1997). In view of these issues the Audit Commission (1992a) underlined the dilemma of home visiting, citing especially patient appreciation versus cost arguments. The Audit Commission researchers recommended

that practitioners carefully target their home visits, and consider clinic attendance and other options such as telephone consultations as alternatives. The
Audit Commission staff calculated that matching travelling time to 'best
practice' localities in England released the equivalent of 400 WTE community practitioners nationwide. Clearly, practice is changing because more
recent Audit Commission (1999) data showed that district nurses saw up to
a third of their patients in clinics, increasingly during out-of-hours sessions
(CBC 1997). On the downside, a PCT manager in the author's study reported that almost one in three patients did not attend (DNAs) their clinic
appointments. If numbers attending clinics were small anyway, DNAs wasted
valuable time. Conversely, if 'no access' home visits were not an issue then
home visits, despite travelling time and cost, could be more efficient than
clinic-based services, especially for residents in deprived areas where car ownership is lower (Audit Commission 1999). As an adjunct, Andrews (2004)
recommended that managers moved clinic-based services to geographical
hot spots, which not only improves access but also practitioner efficiency.

Traffic congestion and charging are growing issues in urban centres and
these too influence service efficiency and effectiveness. Managers and workforce planners are being forced to consider a wide range of patient contact
issues, e.g. the case study PCT in Table 3.8 is a densely populated urban centre, which no doubt reduces travel time although traffic congestion at peak
times increases the time spent in cars. The PCT has one of the lowest car
ownership populations in the country, which may inhibit patients from travelling to surgeries and health centres. Clearly, these are important
workforce-planning considerations.

# Public health

Social, economic and environmental factors are major contributors to good
and poor health. The Royal College of Nursing (RCN 1994) characterized
public health as prolonging life by preventing disease and promoting health.
Community practitioners rely heavily on their understanding of morbidity,
mortality, socioeconomic and other data connected to public health. These
data enable them to focus on individuals and groups at risk, such as those living in deprived areas, and to work closely with hard-to-reach groups in a
multi-agency and cross-boundary way (Chalmers and Kristajanson 1989;
DoH 2001b). They are able to respond to health inequalities, which helps
PCT managers and practitioners improve health. It is hardly surprising therefore that *Liberating the Talents* (DoH 2002c) recommended public health as
the third mainstream activity for community practitioners.

Strengthening community practitioners' public health role is discussed
regularly in the literature, e.g. Bryar (1994) and Chalmers and Kristajanson

(1989) felt that community practitioners with a public health background influence health gain at individual, family and community levels. Moreover, public health nurses work in well-defined geographical areas about which they are knowledgeable. They are trusted by community patients and, therefore, are well placed to use their knowledge, skills and relationships to identify people at risk and to meet their health needs (Hyde 2001).

Billingham (1991), Craig and Smith (1998), Chalmers and Kristajanson (1989), Hyde (2001) and the RCN (1994) envisaged broad public health intervention roles for community practitioners:

- Education: a voluntary change in attitudes using teaching and learning to prevent, for example, coronary heart disease.
- Engineering: technical actions that reduce risk and enable social and environmental change.
- Enforcement: mandatory services designed to improve health.

Consequently, actions by community staff undertaking these roles will be at the individual, group, policy or national level. The ideal local work includes (Craig and Smith 1998; Elliott et al. 2004):

- screening
- health risk assessment
- parenting classes including breast-feeding
- prevention sessions
- counselling and health education sessions
- social and behaviour skills training
- self-worth and self-esteem sessions
- problem-solving classes
- stress management activities
- assertiveness training
- nutrition and exercise sessions
- first aid and accident prevention.

Often these activities are done simultaneously and examples of good practice can be found in the literature, e.g. staff at the Strelley Nursing Development Unit implemented first aid courses for individuals and tackled accident black spots at the community level, while addressing welfare rights at higher levels (RCN 1994).

Chalmers and Kristajanson (1989) underlined the workforce planning and development actions needed to prepare practitioners for public health roles including health education and disease prevention work. Hyde (2001) and Plews et al. (2000), on the other hand, suspected that practitioners were not ready for planning, implementing and evaluating public health projects as a result of traditional primary and community care roles, scarce time, knowledge and skills deficits. The last, according to Plews et al. (2000, p. 9), can be corrected by re-designing curricula, making them interprofessional, intersectorial and evidence based:

> Politically and professionally the principles and practice of public health are currently firmly on the agenda. Public health nursing isn't new. However, the present climate provides an opportunity to further develop the role and services that legitimise and encourage such work . . . there are varying interpretations of public health nursing, lack of collaboration between and within organisations and discipline and limitations in knowledge and skills possessed by practitioners. These issues all present barriers to the development of public health nursing and need to be considered as a matter of urgency if organisations and clinicians are to make the most of current opportunities.

Historically, changing public health work has been difficult as a result of entrenched professional views, separate education and training, and less than satisfactory teamwork (Turton 1985). Large caseload, lack of managerial support, and crisis and reactive work such as child protection are other barriers (Hyde 2001). Hyde (2001) ranked (most to least) the public health activities carried out by practitioners, which highlights other problems:

- Health education
- Illness and accident prevention
- Policy interpretation
- Health promotion
- Empowerment.

These rankings were uniform across different localities but time spent on them varied tenfold. Health visitors and district nurses, despite their low cost and the medical bridge between GPs and public health doctors that they provide (Craig and Smith 1998), were some of the least active public health practitioners. In the past, monitoring the effects of actions to relieve health inequalities has been difficult to enact and evaluate. However, Lewis (2003b) believed that public health is changing and opportunities are increasing.

Poverty is an accepted determinant of poor health, which often goes hand in hand with inequality. Tackling the root causes – substandard housing, poor scholastic achievement, unemployment, lifestyle issues and pollution – are major health determinants (Hyde 2001). Lower socioeconomic classes suffer unequal opportunity and access to health services – the so-called inverse care law where the service distribution is unequal and where practitioners have failed to meet the extra needs of those in deprived areas. Consequently, the World Health Organization (WHO) set 21 public health targets for health service managers, practitioners and policy makers, which can be condensed into four themes (Hyde 2001):

1. Equity
2. Health public policies
3. Multisectorial responsibility for health
4. Lifespan orientation.

However, there are data that reject the inverse care law, e.g. families in deprived areas averaged 14 visits whereas those in the control group received 5.5 visits from health visitors (Rowe et al. 1995). In the UK, health visitors have worked with deprived populations for many years, trying to address the needs of vulnerable groups while at the same time providing a universal service to all families with children aged under 5 (Tudor-Hart 1971; Almond 2002). Public health work, fairly allocated or not, is largely attributed to health visitors because of their principal roles:

• assessing health needs
• stimulating health awareness
• influencing policy that affects health
• facilitating activities that enhance health.

However, Hyde (2001) and Craig and Smith (1998) describe two polemical views of health visiting. First is their pivotal role in primary care which relates to the new public health movement, focusing on health inequalities and health promotion – largely unrecognized in the biomedical model of health care. Health visitors have a range of skills that cover individuals and communities, which depends on PCT commissioning. The second, considerably more negative, view is that public health nursing means that health visiting core functions are disintegrating. There are arguments that health visitor roles are being eroded and usurped by practice nurses. Health visitors bemoan these changes, particularly their colleagues who fail to recognize health visiting knowledge and skills and the long-term contact that they have with patients. Their holistic view of patients – ill, well, in clinics or in the patient's home – is not appreciated. In short, threatened, undervalued and squeezed out, it is hardly surprising that health visitors are one staff group most resistant to delegating work (Wiles and Robinson 1994; Hyde 2001).

As discussed elsewhere, the proportion of 0–15 year olds in PCT populations ranges from 16% to 25%, which is decreasing or growing anywhere from –0.8% to +1.3%. Child-centred activities, as might be expected, predominate in health visiting. Unfortunately, health visitors in some localities, as a result of the medicolegal implications of child protection, spend more time on caseload management and related administration than they do on physical or psychosocial care. Elsewhere, the reverse is true and it is probable that information management and technology (IM&T) and administrative support differences between the sites explain these findings.

A meta-analysis of health visiting activity literature summarizes how practitioners spend their time (Audit Commission 1994; Crofts et al. 2000; Ebeid
2000):

- Direct patient care: 40%
- Indirect care: 25%
- Administrative and clerical: 25–30%
- Travel: 5%.

The large amount of time health visitors spend on paperwork (up to a
third) tends to make these practitioners the most studied and the ones to
come under closest scrutiny (see, for example, Elkan et al. 2000a, 2000b,
2000c). However, they carry out a broad range of work for diverse and sometimes vulnerable groups such as homeless and disadvantaged individuals.
Despite the 'no right of access' and the unsolicited nature of their services,
health visitors are well accepted by patients. Moreover, their universal, home-
centred service means that vulnerable children are not stigmatized,
something that could easily happen with other child-focused services such as
school nursing and social work (Appleton 1994). Health visitors are acutely
aware of this delicate relationship and the length of time these relationships
take to develop (Ledger 1987; Cowley 1995).

Bowns et al.'s (2000) study of 302 mothers is interesting:

- 61% had seen their health visitor in the previous 6 weeks
- 75% had seen her or him in the past 8 weeks
- 7% had never seen a health visitor.
- 43% of the contacts were 9-month reviews, 19% of visits were for weighing
  babies, 14% for advice and 12% for hearing tests.

There has been a significant change in the location of health visitor work
in recent times. Wiseman's (1982a, 1982b) 20-year survey showed that
home visits accounted for 84% of activity. A later report by the CBC (1997),
on the other hand, showed that 54% of health visitor contacts took place in
patients' homes and 37% in clinics. Crofts et al.'s (2000) data were similar
in that home visits accounted for 51% of the caseload, of which 69% were
deemed high priority. The 20-minute average contact seemed to be unrelated to priority.

Health visiting activity has unusual features in that 'no access' was the
third most frequent activity in all 3 years of one large data-set studied by the
author. Dobby and Barnes' (1987a) work showed that 71% of the health visitors' patients ($n$ = 265) required a visit but up to 58% were 'no access' – a 41%
increase since Wiseman's (1982a) study. Dobby and Barnes estimated, for
efficiency and effectiveness, that health visitors needed to visit between nine
and fourteen patients each day to make home visiting worthwhile. However,

Clark (1984) warned that shifting consultations to clinics could be counter-productive because poor facilities, lack of continuity and queuing caused dissatisfaction among mothers. Moreover, as raised earlier, up to 45% of families in some PCT areas do not have use of a car, which influences both clinic attendance and possibly patient satisfaction.

Steele et al.'s (2001) systematic review shows that health visitors make a difference among families living in social adversity. They help to reduce health inequalities while improving long-term health prospects. There are strong arguments for concentrating health-visiting services in deprived areas. Oddly, however, Colliety's (1988a, 1998b) data show that health visitors would not be the first or even the second person mothers would ask for advice. Mothers understood health visiting but as their children grew they were less likely to call on health visitors for advice. Clark (1984) felt that altering access and types of services offered to mothers, such as an out-of-hours crying baby service, could reverse this pattern.

Appleton's work (1994) showed that the relationship between frequency and need varied widely. Between 50% and 80% of health visitors' work was spent with children whereas 35% concentrated on mothers. Elkan et al.'s (2000a, 2000b, 2000c), Coupland's (1986) and Ledger's (1987) evidence underlined the importance of health visitors' work with elderly people, particularly health education, injury prevention, care coordination and unmet need identification. However, Crofts' work showed that elderly care activity barely registered (0.01%). If Crofts' analysis is typical then it is unlikely that health visitors are making a contribution to the 150 elderly surveillance assessments needed in a typical practice each year. However, falling elderly care may not be the health visitors' fault. Specialist elderly care teams, which can include health visitors, are probably usurping the health visitor's role (Fitton 1984a).

Health visitors are autonomous and isolated workers. Some argue that a lack of clarity and purpose contributes to the latter. A more likely explanation, on the other hand, is the way health visitors are deployed and their geographical separation, which can prevent them from taking a wider community perspective. Their reactive and sometimes crisis-oriented work also detracts from wider public health work (Smith 2004). Policy and practice based on health needs assessment are less likely to bear fruit when practitioners are deployed geographically.

Health visitors are accused of ritualized practice but they prioritize work appropriately during staff shortages. Unfortunately, work at these times becomes task oriented rather than holistic family care (Ledger 1987). Kendall and Lissauser (2002) blamed NHS traditions, which they felt are a barrier to flexible working whereas the Audit Commission (1994), Elkan et al. (2000a, 2000b, 2000c) and Hyde (2001) indicated that restricting health-visiting interventions to a narrow range is less effective than the broader ones that address multiple needs of individuals and families. However, targeting only those with problems could allow needy individuals to slip through the net. Universal services, on the other hand, probably waste resources but they do reach vulnerable groups who are less likely to access services.

Kelsey and Robinson (1999) felt that screening of all pre-school children is inefficient and ineffective. A conservative estimate is that 10% of the health visitor's workload is general screening – the equivalent of 1300 WTEs at a cost of £26m. Consequently, questions are often asked about cost-effectiveness. However, there are arguments that routine screening opportunities provided by hearing and sight tests could, for example, unearth child abuse cases (Kendrick et al. 1995; Kelsey and Robinson 1999). However, authors bemoan the lack of evidence that help managers make decisions about routine screening or targeted services. Helpfully, Audit Commission (1994) researchers recommended that all families with new babies should be visited. Thereafter, visits to the same family should be prioritized and based on need. One advantage of this approach is that health visitors could practise flexibly: family centred, crisis oriented, universally or targeted depending on the context (Smith 2004).

## Other public health workers

School nurses have an important public health role. However, Cotton et al. (2000) feel that these practitioners are increasingly out of step and could be more efficiently and effectively employed if they target needy children rather than trying to provide a blanket service (a similar argument to health visiting work). School nursing activity in Cotton et al.'s study from most to least is shown in Table 3.9.

**Table 3.9** School nursing activity in study of Cotton et al. (2000)

| Activity | Time spent (%)[a] |
|---|---|
| Screening | 60 (20) |
| Health promotion | 22 (23) |
| Child protection | 6.6 (4.5) |
| Immunization | 4 (3) |
| Drop-in sessions | 3.8 (3.2) |

[a] Values in parentheses are the standard deviation (SD).

Looking after children with special needs and teenage pregnancy barely registered in Cotton et al.'s (2000) study. Things may be changing because despite these activity data, few practitioners in Cotton et al.'s survey wanted to continue routine screening, preferring instead targeted health promotion services and open-access advisory sessions, the second and last activity in the study. Unlike earlier fieldwork, deprivation was the main dependent variable driving school nursing activity – explaining 24% of the variance. However, there was no significant association with any other social or economic variable such as special needs and child protection. Cotton et al. (2000) recommended that PCT commissioners needed to double their spending on school nursing services to bring local services up to their best.

Schools in some of the localities studied by the author were changing their educational status and pupil numbers were expected to increase by 5%. One potential implication of the change/rise is the way the teenage pregnancy strategy is interpreted and applied (DoH 2001b), e.g. as a result of a high incidence of pregnant teenagers addicted to drugs, managers said that health visitors, social service staff, family planning and school nurses were working together. Consequently, roles were blurring and 'one-stop shops' were a possibility. It seems that the Future Healthcare Workforce prophecies (Conrane Consulting et al. 1999) are slowly being realized.

Other community nurses are also well placed to undertake public health work, particularly when there is a risk that district nurses are seen as mainly CDM workers. However, district nursing is largely a 'referred to' service – a way of rationing primary and community care. If district nurses are to be more involved in public health and in preventing those in need slipping through the net, more resources will be needed especially in PCTs that are stretched (Hyde 2001).

Issues about closer working with social services are important not only because partnerships between health and social care are expected to benefit health-care efficiency and effectiveness but also because of the common problems faced by health and social care professionals – especially when dealing with young people. Interviewees in the author's study welcomed joint working because duplication by health and social carers can be reduced. Schemes introduced recently by the Department of Health (2001b) were often described by interviewees. These were expected to improve health and social care, and influence joint working. Policy initiatives for the young, such as Sure Start, is one example. As elsewhere, although laudable and supported by managers and practitioners, no interviewee was clear how the workload implications of new initiatives such as Children's Trusts would be handled (Hyde 2001). One PCT manager felt that child welfare was particularly demanding but demand can fluctuate (Table 3.10).

In one PCT studied by the author, child protection registrations had increased by 35% in 1 year whereas other PCTs had seen a 40% fall. Managers perceived that demand for community practitioner services was being increased by families and children in their areas because family stressors were rising and that 'looked after' children were steadily joining practitioners' caseloads. These issues were compounded because homes

**Table 3.10** Demand for child welfare

| PCT/Band | < 6 years (%) | 6–15 years (%) | Lone parent (%) | Child protection registration (%) |
|---|---|---|---|---|
| England | 5.9 | 14.3 | 5.8 | 0.04 |
| Three-star PCTs | 5.6 | 14.4 | 5.7 | 0.05 |
| ONS Band 1 PCTs | 6.6 | 12.2 | 8.2 | 0.07 |
| ONS Band 2 | 5.8 | 14.7 | 7.4 | 0.05 |
| ONS Band 3 | 6.1 | 14.8 | 7.5 | 0.02 |
| ONS Band 4 | 5.7 | 13.9 | 6.1 | 0.05 |
| ONS Band 5 | 6.1 | 14.3 | 5 | 0.04 |
| ONS Band 6 | 5.5 | 13.9 | 5.5 | 0.06 |
| Specimen Band 3 PCT | 5.8 | 14 | 9.9 | 0.1 |
| PCT's percentile | 45th | 42nd | 98th | 100th |

were visited rather than parents and children attending clinics (CBC 1997). Therefore, managers in PCTs with younger populations in areas of high deprivation were likely to be more or less stretched operationally and strategically.

As a result of this complex and complicated picture, Ebeid (2000) believed that practitioners increasingly were being asked to demonstrate value for money and to meet rising demand. They were expected to show their unique skills while working to evidence-based protocols. They should also take the opportunity to manage and lead health-care teams. Hyde (2001), on the other hand, is worried that public health nursing is ad hoc and marginal and that a more strategic approach is required. Options include specialist practitioners who work alongside caseload-holding colleagues, thereby separating the public health function from generic/universal roles or, alternatively, a generic, multiskilled practitioner, who works alongside GPs at the centre of primary health care. There is a risk, however, that adding another staff category may fragment primary and community care further. Coalescence of existing jobs may be the compromise solution.

The Department of Health emphasizes a multidisciplinary public health workforce. Professional clarity and direction about interagency working is, however, needed and multidisciplinary teamwork has to be coordinated. Leaders have to motivate, innovate and develop new public health services (DoH 2001b). It is anticipated that public health nurses such as health visitors will make a significant contribution to this work, although there are worries that health visitors do not have the time and in some cases the knowledge and skills to take on a wider public health role (Denny 1989; DoH 1993c; Smith 2004). Smith (2004) explained that the breadth and depth of current primary and community workers' roles influence perceptions of what public health work means. Consequently, both Smith (2004) and Hyde (2001) explore ways in which the traditional primary health-care team can be developed for public health work. Local public health leaders may help public health departments and unrelated staff such as health visitors by 'bringing practitioners in from the cold'. In short, formal networks are needed.

## Productivity

Productivity as an aspect of workforce planning can be discussed only under the traditional primary and community care roles because contact data are geared along the same lines (and will not be recorded in the future anyway). Nevertheless, district nurses follow up 80% of the patients referred to them within 24 hours (Audit Commission 1999). District nurses in one PCT studied by the author handle large caseloads, which makes the 24-hour follow-up standard even more impressive. These anecdotal data are corroborated by a broader study, which also showed that high proportions of patients spend protracted time in the care of district nurses (Audit Commission 1999). Consequently, Dewis (2001) analysed the length of time patients spent 'on the books' (Table 3.11).

**Table 3.11** Time patients spend 'on the books'

| Time (months) | Percentage |
| --- | --- |
| 48+ | 15 |
| 18–24 | 14 |
| 6–12 | 14 |
| 1–3 | 10 |
| 24–36 | 10 |
| 36–48 | 9 |
| 0–3 | 5 |

Dewis's (2001) analysis also revealed the frequency of district nurse visits (Table 3.12).

**Table 3.12** Frequency of district nurse visits

| Visit frequency | Percentage |
| --- | --- |
| Six monthly | 55 |
| Three monthly | 10 |
| Weekly | 10 |
| Bi-weekly | 8 |
| Monthly | 5 |
| Daily | 5 |

Unsurprisingly, the greater a practitioner's caseload the less frequently each patient is visited ($r_s$ = 0.62) (Audit Commission 1999). Almost one in five patients on district nursing caseloads are visited at least weekly (Audit Commission's 1999; Dewis 2001). This finding supports the argument that district nursing interventions are largely supervisory and pastoral.

Hyatt (2003) felt that long-term vacancies (officially 3 months) create a 'workaholic' mentality among many community staff. These workers felt that there was never enough time and that their services fell short of the ideals that they and others held. Analysis of their caseloads revealed efficiency (doing things right) but not effectiveness (doing the right things). Productivity and crisis management were linked with practitioners tending to cope and reorganize care without systematically documenting the cause or effects (Goodman 1996). Strategic and operational planning suffered and staff became discouraged and passive. Although the data are old, Goldstone and Worral (1980) showed that overstaffed community teams were characterized by low direct care and travelling times whereas other staff spent more time in their health centres and had longer meal breaks. Hyatt (2003) also showed that equitably staffed health-visiting teams worked more appropriately. Understaffed localities and families with social problems, on the other hand, seem to restrict health visitors' roles.

The controversial NHS Executive value for money (VFM) study (Cowley 1993; Goodman 1996) showed that community teams were top heavy and worked inappropriately. The authors criticized the amount of time practitioners spent communicating, implying that this work was low value. The VFM team was criticized for de-emphasizing community nurses' caseload management, coordination and liaison work, which increased the amount of time practitioners spent communicating. The nature and value of communication are not easily measured and may not feature in any process or outcome data, which is bound to influence employers' perceptions (Elkan et al. 2000a, 2000b, 2000c). In contrast, immunization work has clear targets and clear incentives, and is well coordinated and successful (Audit Commission 1994). Table 3.13, which summarizes activity data from 24 health authorities, shows why some independent observers are concerned.

**Table 3.13** Staff activity by professional group (McDonald et al. 1997)

| Activity | District nurse (%) | Health visitor (%) | School nurse (%) |
| --- | --- | --- | --- |
| Patient contact | 47–85 | 7–44 | 0–60 |
| Classroom/clinics | 0–2 | 8–19 | 12–55 |
| Patient related | 0–19 | 14–40 | 0–30 |
| Administration | 5–22 | 1–24 | 5–42 |
| Travel | 0–16 | 4–13 | 2–13 |
| Other | 0–30 | 0–19 | 0–34 |

These data are remarkably robust because other studies showed that community practitioners spend anywhere between 45% and 83% of their time in direct patient care (Audit Commission 1992a). The inverse relationship between seniority and direct care noted in hospital nursing activity (Hurst 2003) seems to apply equally to the community sector. District nurses, for example, can spend up to 68% of their time in administrative work (Audit Commission 1999) and managers rightly question whether these nurses are working efficiently and effectively.

As can be seen in Table 3.14, district nursing, health visiting and assistant health practitioner (AHP) activity data vary widely.

**Table 3.14** Number of patient contacts per practitioner

| PCT/Band | Health visitors | District nurses | Podiatrists | Occupational therapists | Physio-therapists |
|---|---|---|---|---|---|
| England | 1356 | 395 | 1034 | 83 | 296 |
| Three-star PCTs | 1193 | 405 | 937 | 112 | 337 |
| ONS Band 1 PCTs | 1185 | 354 | 687 | Not available | 296 |
| ONS Band 2 | 1553 | 648 | 921 | 85 | 217 |
| ONS Band 3 | 1055 | 783 | 1156 | 131 | 334 |
| ONS Band 4 | 1535 | 365 | 967 | 79 | 296 |
| ONS Band 5 | 1580 | 310 | 1127 | 79 | 290 |
| ONS Band 6 | 1234 | 451 | 1067 | 103 | 330 |
| Specimen Band 3 PCT | 709 | 1248 | NA | NA | NA |
| PCT's percentile | 10th | 98th | | | |

NA, not applicable.

Higher productivity not only has workload and staffing but also recruitment and retention implications. It has to be questioned whether higher activity levels can be sustained and are, therefore, equitable. However, with the exception of some specialist practitioners, the number of patient contacts in England is falling (Audit Commission 1999; DoH 2002c). Two and three-quarter million patients receive care from district nurses every year, which equates to 36 million contacts. However, these are falling yearly by 4–6%. Nevertheless, 5% of the population will have contact with community staff each year. Half of those aged over 85 year are seen by a district nurse, and their numbers are growing.

As discussed earlier, there are concerns in the literature about the nature and value of school nursing interventions. Some practitioners were active in areas unrelated to need and poorly rationalized, and their effectiveness unmeasured (Audit Commission 1994). Consequently, Audit Commission staff suggested that practitioners' knowledge and skills were under-used and recommended that work should be targeted, thought of as either 'universal' such as immunization, child health surveillance and sex education, or 'selective support' such as child protection and care of looked-after children. Gleeson (2003) underlined the opportunity practitioners have when dealing with teenagers' health – at the forefront of many government agendas. They are at considerable risk of ill-health from smoking, substance misuse and sexually transmitted disease. Moreover, teenagers are reluctant to approach GPs (less so nurses) as a result of confidentiality issues, embarrassment and a lack of sympathy. Approachable, same-sex staff, confidential consulting rooms and drop-in sessions are likely to ease teenagers' perceived problems.

Specialist community practitioner activity is mixed. Macmillan nurse contacts at 60 000 per year are rising whereas Marie Curie practitioner activity fell by 11%. Continence adviser contacts increased by 40%, outstripped by community paediatric nurse activity which doubled. The contact of practitioners who specialize in diabetes rose 18% and sexual health practitioner work also increased steadily as a result of recently implemented flexible service times and drop-in sessions. Health visitor contacts rose steadily until 1997, but since then there has been a 1% per year reduction. School nurse data are not collected centrally. However, manager interviewees in the author's study perceived that workload was rising to the extent that practitioners are beginning to work during school holidays.

Turning to allied health professionals, podiatrists' activities, as one might expect, consisted largely of basic and technical foot care. Since 1998, the number of contacts fell by 3% a year after a 13% increase in the decade to 1998. However, the NSF for Diabetes is expected to reverse this trend. Occupational therapy contacts continue to rise from 1% to 8% annually. Typically, the number of contacts in occupational therapy is 44 per 1000 population, which has been increasing by 8% per year as a result of step-down care and outreach work. Physiotherapy contacts rose dramatically (35%) in the first part of the last decade, but recently the number has stabilized. Analysis of physiotherapy activity in one PCT showed that staff easily exceeded the Chartered Society of Physiotherapy's (CSP's) benchmarks. One reason for this level of activity is that the number of referrals from GPs to therapy services is increasing steadily over time (ACPM/CSP 2002).

Speech and language therapy (SaLT) activity data are not collected centrally but SaLT activity in the case study sites showed that 'documentation' activities were steadily rising probably for medicolegal reasons. Managers' perceptions were that SaLT activity increased because roles were extending. Dietetic staff activity is collected centrally and has changed over time. Practitioners' interventions continue to focus on assessing patients and evaluating progress. Occupational therapists' interventions fluctuated over time. Nevertheless, therapists are activities of daily living (ADL) oriented, especially mobility-focused interventions. Therapists in one PCT studied by the author recorded more managerial and administrative activities than their counterparts in other PCTs.

Managers and practitioners are incredulous about central databases that show falling contact because they do not match perceptions, e.g. one manager's data showed that referrals were outstripping discharges largely because of the NSFs. One interviewee's referral increases were entirely GP based. Another manager, less vulnerable to referrals, showed that her increasing activity was generated by extra evening clinics that better suited her patients. One manager raised an interesting observation – the contact drop-off coincided with the transfer from manual Kalamazoo recording systems to electronic collection and storage of activity data, which may mean that electronic data recording is not as complete or as accurate as manual recording systems. On the other hand, an equally plausible explanation for falling contacts is, as discussed earlier, the shifting (notably evening) work from community to social services (Audit Commission 1999).

## Time out

Time out is shorthand for authorized and unauthorized absence. Typically, the NHS time out average is 22%, i.e. more than one practitioner in five is away from work at any time. At first glance, therefore, establishments are less generous than they first appear. The one-in-five rule, although sobering, is generally not appreciated by managers and workforce planners. The sickness absence part of time out is collected centrally, which shows a two-and-a-half times difference between the lowest and highest PCT (Table 3.15).

**Table 3.15** Sickness absence levels

| PCT/Band | Sickness (%) | Job satisfaction |
|---|---|---|
| England | 4.1 | 3[a] |
| Three-star PCTs | 4 | 3 |
| ONS Band 1 PCTs | 4.5 | 3 |
| ONS Band 2 | 4.3 | 3 |
| ONS Band 3 | 4.1 | 3 |
| ONS Band 4 | 4.2 | 3 |
| ONS Band 5 | 3.7 | 3 |
| ONS Band 6 | 4.2 | 3 |
| Specimen Band 3 PCT | 2.3 | 3 |
| PCT's percentile | 7th | NA |

[a] 5 is the highest rating.

Ten years ago, NHS staff took less leave than the Confederation of British Industry time-out average and considerably less than the public sector average (Anonymous 1994). However, recent data show that NHS sickness is greater than public services generally – an interesting reversal. Managers admitted in their interviews that they struggled continuously with short- and long-term sick leave especially when professional teams were small. A vicious cycle was emerging: under-staffing led to work pressures that led to sickness, which led to under-staffing. Local data indicated that community practitioner sick leave was more likely to be workload and stress related.

District nurses have the highest sickness rate of all the primary and community professionals. However, 15% of district nurses' sick leave was injury based, whereas 8% took work-related time out (the same proportion as the nursing profession generally). Soberingly and worryingly, up to 40% of district nurses' absence was injury or work related – equivalent to an average of 8 days per practitioner per year. Time out varied between staff, e.g. 3% took 75 or more days leave per year (Anonymous 1994, p. 10):

> District nurses are a loyal workforce, with the majority taking little or no sickness-absence. The study indicates, however, that working conditions are far from satisfactory, that employees are being exposed to continued risk to their physical and mental health and safety at work, and that many are suffering from work-related health problems, which leads to significant lost time.

Recent data showed that sickness absence among front-line staff, such as general practitioner receptionists, was growing especially among those facing the general public and who find it more difficult to 'move away from the desk'. However, time out is a complex issue and an important problem for managers to solve in view of recruitment and retention problems and the bank, agency and overtime costs that they face. Allen (2001) suggests novel but effective solutions such as confidential counselling service for front-line staff.

## Conclusion

How primary and community care practitioners spend their time is important for:

- estimating staff numbers and mix
- ensuring equitable workloads
- evaluating efficiency and effectiveness.

These data offer valuable insights into workload, working styles, job satisfaction, recruitment, retention and outcomes. Staff activity and performance data in the literature (see Annotated bibliography, page 167) and the national databases are becoming increasingly accessible and usable. However, data can sometimes require considerable unravelling before they make sense. In some cases data are confusing because they reflect the different ways that work activities were classified, collected and recorded. Consequently, strenuous efforts have been made to standardize the data in this book to help managers benchmark their localities.

Even then, primary and community care WP&D is a complex and challenging area not least because activity data are conflicting, e.g. community patient dependency and acuity are increasing, whereas the numbers of community patient contacts among some professional groups are falling annually, anywhere from 1% to 11%. Moreover, the PCT WP&D database shows that some practitioners are twice as 'productive' as colleagues in the same ONS Band. Specialist practitioner (such as community paediatric nurses) contacts are rising dramatically – doubling in some cases. Consequently, community practitioner activities need to be scrutinized and monitored by managers and practitioners because basing staffing on average activity data alone would be unfair and inequitable.

Working styles fluctuate greatly between different PCTs and over time. Indeed, evidence shows that primary and community staff lean towards indirect care and administrative work probably for medicolegal reasons – the maxim 'if it's not recorded then it's not done' is a powerful record-keeping driver. Understandably, managers are worried that direct patient care takes second place to administrative work – up to 42% of practitioners' time. Another managerial concern is that some PCTs have generous numbers of administrative staff per head of population so managers should explore the level of clerical (and IM&T) support given to clinical staff.

Travelling, no access and patient non-attendance at clinics also continue to be negative issues in the literature. Consequently, staff can spend a quarter of their working day on travel to patients' homes and clinics which does not bear fruit (no access or DNAs). However, the situation is complex and managers need to consider a range of variables including population density, traffic congestion, geographical working and household car ownership before adjusting working styles and care locations, e.g. a PCT with proportionally more deprivation, including residents without independent transport, can expect higher clinic non-attendance data.

Time out, not always fully appreciated by managers, especially workload-related short and long sick leave, is a continuous struggle for PCT managers because sick leave erodes budgets. Indeed, the sickness absence rate in some PCTs is double the ONS Band average in which they sit. Based on the average PCT establishment, an extra 1% sickness rate alone means an additional 10 absent WTEs. Clearly, time out is an area that needs investigating when the cause is related to work injury or stress.

New and important Modernisation and Changing Workforce programmes are likely to cause managers to rethink staff activity. The core functions of *Liberating the Talents* (LtT) (DoH 2002c) and Evercare, for example, are emerging as the activities most likely to influence the size and mix of primary and community teams. However, managers will be hampered because staff activity data are organized along traditional workforce lines, whereas LtT and Evercare core functions are patient centred and interdisciplinary. Nevertheless, traditional PCT WP&D data still have value for reconfiguring PCT workforces. Another tension facing managers is the contradiction between the staggering rise in specialist practitioner contacts (such as nurses with special interests like diabetes mellitus) and arguments for generic, multiskilled workers in the literature, particularly when efficiency and effectiveness are not issues.

One LtT category, First Contact, concerns several members of the primary and community care teams. Demand for primary care services is rising and there is a shortage of GPs. The number of practice nurses per head of population is double in some PCTs, which is inversely related to the number of GPs. These outcomes mean that nurses' primary care first contact responsibilities are likely to increase – a role for which they are well suited. As a result of PMS and the new GMS contract issues, PCT managers with diluted practice nursing workforces may need to consider boosting practice nurse numbers or widen practitioner job descriptions to cover primary care first contact work. There are barriers to developing first contact work, notably sickness certification, nurse prescribing limitations and professional resistance, which policy makers and PCT managers need to overcome. These barriers interfere with 24- and 48-hour access performance, which vary up to 30% in the PCT WP&D database. Access to primary care services is sensitive not only to primary care staffing but also to extended roles.

Chronic disease management, continuing care and rehabilitation in the community are the second LtT core function. As with First Contact work, demand is increasing because of an ageing population, changing morbidity and shifting of secondary to primary care. However, if the number of patient contacts is a measure of demand then the picture is confused because patient contact with some professionals has fallen by 11% in recent years. Transfer of community nursing work to Social Services is the probable explanation although the number of unpaid carer hours has increased disproportionately in some PCTs. However, Social Service care does not fully explain a fourfold variation in the number of patient–practitioner contacts in the PCT WP&D database. These outputs, important for equity, recruitment and retention reasons, are explored later.

Referrals to community practitioners are likely to continue rising and the issues that influence referrals vary widely. However, four categories of inappropriate referral persist, which waste practitioners' time and skills:

1. The patient was referred to the wrong practitioner.
2. The patient was inappropriately discharged.

3. The patient did not need care.
4. The patient referral led to duplicated work.

There is disagreement in the literature about the number of inappropriate referrals to community nurses, which have efficiency, effectiveness and job satisfaction implications. Concern about community nurses' pastoral role, on the other hand, has diminished because:

• monitoring visits help to maintain elderly patients in the community
• the contributions from unpaid carers are rising – individuals who need support and a professional contact.

Public health nursing, the third *Liberating the Talents* core function, is expected to influence the way a range of primary care staff work, notably health visitors and school nurses. The number of these practitioners per head of a PCT population varies remarkably – almost double in the case of health visitors in some PCTs. Managers are interested in these data for equitable staffing, recruitment and retention, and cost and quality reasons.

Public health interventions are being aimed at health inequality, especially deprived areas with under-served residents – a sector in which public health practitioners can make a great difference. However, as staffing and productivity fluctuate widely, decisions about whether public health becomes subsumed into existing job descriptions or, on the other hand, part of a specialist practitioner's role are unresolved. There is support for both approaches but, if public health is to become routine in a range of community practitioners' work, then elderly care may need to feature more in the routine work of all practitioners. Universal versus targeted contact and the duplication arising from the overlap between health and social care child welfare services also need to be considered by managers. All these have staff education and training implications.

The number of allied health professional contacts in the community fluctuates but is growing steadily. The NSFs are expected to raise community demand for these services. These issues at least will cause PCT managers to reconsider multidisciplinary and interdisciplinary work in the community.

# CHAPTER FOUR

# Staff mix

## Introduction and background

Skill mix is defined as the balance of trained and untrained, qualified and unqualified, registered and unregistered, supervisory and operative staff, and proportions of workers in different staff groups in distinct areas. Grade mix, on the other hand, relates to staff grades, their activities and costs. An alternative definition is to think of grade mix as *intraprofessional* and skill mix as *interprofessional* (Richards et al. 2000; Wright 1998). Somewhat cynically, Rink et al. (1996) perceive grade mix as a method of reducing costs whereas skill mix is about balancing relevant qualifications, skills and experience to meet local community patients' needs.

Grade mix and skill mix are phrases that are often used interchangeably by workforce planners and developers, but as the definitions above imply they are different. The more preferable universal phrase 'staff mix' covers both skill and grade mix and is a less emotive phrase (Medical Practices Committee or MPC 2001, p. 4):

> [staff mix is] the use of a variety of professionals, with varying qualities and expertise, to carry out roles traditionally performed by one healthcare professional. Carried to its extreme, the theory is that all staff should be working to their maximum potential at all times.

The Department of Health (DoH 2001b, pp. 32–33) stresses the relationship between staff mix and a modernized NHS workforce:

> Nearly one million people work for the NHS. They bring a range of skills to bear on treating and caring for patients. They are scarce resources and we need to make the best use of their skills and expertise. And that means, among other things, that we need to have in place good systems for workforce planning and development, which will ensure, so far as we can, that we have sufficient staff available with the right skills to deliver high quality care to patients.

The Department of Health (2001c), corroborating work by Rapport and Maggs (1997), add why recent workforce planning generally and staff mix initiatives specifically have failed:

- Plans not built around service needs and the skills required
- Workforce, service and financial planning poorly integrated
- Workforce planning fragmented, looking separately at primary, community and secondary care and at different staff groups
- Does not include patients' and carers' views
- The plan not responsive to service changes and developments
- Planning poorly supported by the education sector
- As a result of weak connections between staff demand and supply.

To correct these weaknesses, historical approaches and divisions between different groups are being dismantled and replaced with local activities, including those services seen as peripheral to workforce planning and development such as finance. These are needed to make workforce-planning processes centre staged, relevant and worthwhile.

The MPC (2001) and Poulton and West (1994) explain that primary and community care staff-mix reviews are about improving service efficiency and effectiveness, making the best use of resources, matching knowledge and skills to services, and identifying and plugging the gaps. Workforce reviews are also important because of the spectrum, quality and cost of health and social care (Editorial 1997; Wright 1998; Audit Commission 1999; Jenkins-Clarke and Carr-Hill 2001a, 2001b). Inappropriate working by experienced health-care professionals, resulting from staff-mix imbalance, is a national problem. In one study, for example, up to two-thirds of the community workforce felt that their primary care team's mix was inappropriate, which caused them to work ineffectively and inefficiently. Practitioners' biggest gripe, as raised in earlier chapters, was the administrative and clerical burdens placed on them (Wright 1998; Richards et al. 2000).

It is argued in the literature that health-care reforms will not succeed unless both the number and mix of employees are sufficient and appropriate to meet the workload and that primary and community staff are properly educated and managed (Anonymous 1994; Cooper 1997). A recent Department of Health policy document *Making a Difference* describes four levels of worker (Buchan and Edwards 2000):

1. health-care assistant
2. registered practitioner
3. senior registered practitioner
4. consultant practitioner.

The North American Kaiser Permanente organization's staff-mix approach is similar (Craig 2003):

- health and social care assistants
- consultant practitioners
- supervisors.

The more technically skilled registered practitioner is weaker in the latter model – an important role for efficient and effective primary and community care according to the NHS Management Executive value for money (VFM) study (NHS Management Executive 1992). The VFM report authors suggested that the workforce consists of leaders and care managers who assess needs and delegate work to junior staff such as community staff nurses. They also recommended that care assistants be included in the team to support both the leader and the community practitioner. Although the VFM report was heavily criticized in the nursing and other press, Prideaux's (1996) independent work also suggested that the primary and community nursing workforce was district nurse rich and support worker weak.

It is difficult to imagine whether the NHS skill deficit will enhance or counter staff-mix changes (Buchan and Edwards 2000). The question of technical skilled practitioner-dominated care team versus activities of living-based community care assistant can probably be answered only if high-quality, reproducible health needs, dependency–acuity and other data are available to managers (Edwardson and Nardone 1990; Rashid et al. 1996). Ebeid (2000) and MPC (2001), for example, considered the following variables and data when reviewing staff mix in their locality (interestingly, these are a mix of quantitative [hard data] and qualitative [soft data] methods):

- mix of professional qualifications
- extent of post-basic education and training
- staff members' CVs
- practitioners' special interests
- caseloads, especially number of families, children with special needs, child protection, travelling and clinic sessions
- staff safety
- job acceptability and satisfaction.

The good news is that data for many of these variables for each PCT have been collated and made available to the reader in the PCT workforce planning and development (WP&D) database, and are explored in case studies throughout the book.

The recently introduced *Liberating the Talents'* core roles (DoH 2002c) also offer a framework in which to consider primary and community care staff mix:

- First contact
- Continuing care and chronic disease management (CDM)
- Public health.

These core functions are vital to the Department of Health's future workforce intentions and, if realized, may make the traditional staff groups obsolete.

## Grade-mix and skill-mix drivers and restrainers

Staff mix is a sensitive issue as a result of fears about cutbacks and what seems an obvious solution to financial problems because staff costs, at 68–70%, are the largest NHS budget component (Heath 1994; Poulton and West 1994). Saving money by delegating work to lower-grade staff is without doubt an attractive way of saving money. A cheaper service with the same level of activity and to the same level of quality is a tall order, however, e.g. Cowley (1993) argued that top-down (management-led) staff-mix adjustments is reductionist, unholistic and mechanistic and inevitably leads to staff-mix dilution, which seems at odds with the drive to improve NHS quality. Bottom-up, professional and intuitive methods supported by health needs-based methods, on the other hand, lead to a more flexible and not necessarily a more expensive workforce. However, it is clear from the present literature review that empirical evidence for judging these issues is thin, although three-star trusts in the WP&D database are not only better staffed but also richer in registered practitioners.

In short, as a result of changing local and national policy, poorly aligned education and training, professional rivalry and differences, such changes are likely to provide workforce planners with many challenges (McIntosh et al. 2000). Nevertheless, there is plenty of scope in the community and primary care literature for staff-mix adjustments to improve healthcare efficiency and effectiveness (Rodriguez 1994; Jeffreys et al. 1995; Wright 1998).

Authors began discussing inappropriate working as a staff-mix issue 30 years ago (Dalton et al. 1972) and, over the years, several primary and community staffing mix drivers and restrainers have accumulated. Driving forces include the following (Audit Commission 1992a; Bryar 1994; Heath 1994; Rodriguez 1994; Seymour 1994; Jeffreys et al. 1995; Rink et al. 1996; Barret and Hudson 1997; Buckingham and Wilson 1997; Cooper 1997; McDonald et al. 1997; Rapport and Maggs 1997; Syson-Nibbs 1997; Gerrish et al. 1998;

Nicholson 1998; Wright 1998; Davies 2000a, 2000b; Ebeid 2000; McIntosh et al. 2000; Richards et al. 2000; Hyde 2001; Jenkins-Clarke and Carr-Hill 2001a, 2001b; MPC 2001):

- Deprivation, morbidity and mortality patterns that mean services have to be aligned to local health and social care needs.
- Rising community patient dependency and concomitant workload.
- New services such as intermediate care, rapid response teams, peripatetic clinics, home support and respite care.
- Modernization of the workforce by reviewing posts as vacancies arise such as replacing one type of worker with another.
- Multidisciplinary teams that break down professional barriers, which encourage disparate professionals to work together.
- National and local health policies such as Personal Medical Service (PMS), NHS Direct, walk-in centres and the National Service Frameworks (NSFs).
- Reference costs and other financial benchmarks that lead to cost containment by re-grading posts and reducing hours.
- Falling staff morale and job dissatisfaction which lead to recruitment and retention difficulties. Increasing the variety of workers and therefore decreasing the reliance on one professional group can offset recruitment and retention problems.
- Inter- and intra-group delegation.
- Clinician:manager ratios.
- Shifting from secondary to primary and community care.
- Protocol-based working.
- Changing role boundaries and increased opportunities to extend and expand roles. Practitioners are better educated and becoming more confident, which boosts job satisfaction among other things.
- Reducing inappropriate working and inefficiencies, not least duplication by health and Social Service staff.
- Rising patient expectations.

Several barriers to staff-mix changes also emerge from the literature (Cowley 1993; Bryar 1994; Heath 1994; Rodriguez 1994; Rink et al. 1996; Roberts and Anstead 1996; Rapport and Maggs 1997; Gerrish et al. 1998; Ebeid 2000; Richards et al. 2000; Hyde 2001; MPC 2001):

- Fears surrounding hidden agendas to save money and a lack of resources when richer staff mixes are justified.
- Anecdotal and shroud-waving rationales for richer mixes that fail to impress non-clinical managers.
- Nurses encroaching on medical practice and subsequent professional resistance, jealousy and anxiety.
- Loss of nurses' unique role and autonomy. Creating new nurse

handmaiden phenomena as technical work is delegated from medical to
nurse practitioners.
- Tightly defined job descriptions inherited from clinical re-grading exercises, which led to inflexible and task-oriented working. These are felt to
have de-skilled nurses who became disillusioned or hold feelings of being
exploited, which led to refusal to 'act up'.
- Top-down workforce planning that causes middle managers to feel awk-
ward and vulnerable.
- Managers failing to use practitioners' expert knowledge and skills for
determining staff mix when the situation is unpredictable and less clear.
Similarly, failure to acknowledge carer's understanding of the patients'
needs and situation.
- Professional-oriented staff mix rather than a patient needs-led one.
- Staff-mix inconsistencies between PCTs.
- Lack of understanding about professional roles.
- Higher-grade staff reduced to delegators and supervisors which erodes
their clinical role and job satisfaction.
- Conflicting evidence that diluting staff mix does not save money or
reduce the quality of care such as patient satisfaction.
- Protocols/care pathways that allow practitioners to work autonomously
are expensive to create and maintain.
- Skill constraints owing to legal strictures and educational shortcomings.

Each of these drivers and restrainers at some time has influenced staff mix
to a greater or lesser extent (Gibbing 1995; Nicholson 1998), e.g. Barret and
Hudson (1997) showed how nursing activity changed in the 1990s after the
Community Care Act's effect on the workforce, i.e. contrary to the NHS
VFM study, dependency, acuity and activity data showed a greater demand
for qualified practitioners in the community as technical care increased and
basic, personal care activities were transferred to local authority staff.

## Delegation and extended roles

General practitioners delegate a substantial portion of their consultations
and other work to their primary and community care colleagues.
Appropriate delegation means, even at a conservative estimate, that 11–22%
of GPs' time could be saved. However, actual delegation seems irrational.
Researchers showed that between 4% and 17% of GPs' work was delegated
in the UK (34% in North America) whereas 86% had a delegatable element
(80% in North America). Another confounder was that, although 90% of
GPs wanted to see primary health-care team members' roles develop, only
30% felt that these changes were heading in the right direction because of

the following (Editorial 1997; Hirst et al. 1998; Richardson et al. 1998; Jenkins-Clarke and Carr-Hill 2001a, 2001b; MPC 2001; Kendall and Lissauer 2003):

- Professional jealousies and rivalry as GPs' work was being usurped
- Failure to delegate tasks from doctors to nurses because of task complexity
- Patients not accepting nurses
- Worries about work duplication
- Delegating mundane tasks
- Scepticism about nurses' basic and post-basic education and training to undertake delegated work
- Irrational and uneven approaches to delegation.

Nevertheless, pressures and opportunities for GPs to delegate their work are growing (Richardson et al. 1998), although there are unanswered questions:

- Which diagnostic, treatment and referrals should be delegated for efficiency and effectiveness?
- Do non-medical practitioners act as substitutes or do they complement GPs?
- What incentives facilitate these substitutions?

Delegation and role extension go beyond nursing, e.g. there is considerable interest in developing pharmacists' medicine management and CDM roles (Kendall and Lissauer 2003). However, delegation from medical to nurse and other practitioners is strongly associated with extended roles, which is not simply about replacing doctors and higher-grade nurses or saving money, but about other health-care professionals filling vacuums in certain specialist areas. Specially educated and trained nurses, for example, reduce not only GP workloads but also health service costs, and improve the quality of care not least because knowledge and skills are concentrated in fewer hands (Wilson et al. 2002; Kendall and Lissauer 2003). However, there is conflicting evidence such as substitute workers taking longer to complete tasks previously done by higher-grade staff. There are widespread variations in practice in the UK as well as mixed support among medical practitioners for extending roles, e.g. there are problems arising from the 1992 *Scope of Professional Practice* regulations (United Kingdom Central Council for Nursing, Midwifery and Health Visiting or UKCC 1992) such as nurses writing sickness and death certificates, signing prescriptions, referring patients to secondary care or sectioning mentally ill patients. PMS schemes, designed to increase the flexibility of primary care, are constrained because of the legal requirement for patients to be registered with a medical rather than a nurse practitioner. Consequently, some employers, despite recruitment and retention problems, are unwilling to reorganize work. Curiously, extended role is a lesser issue in North America, notwithstanding its more litigious society (Kendall and Lissauer 2003).

# Clinical re-grading

Clinical re-grading introduced a troubled variable into workforce planning and development. The main issue was that identical posts in neighbouring health authorities were graded higher. The Audit Commission (1992a) estimated that generous re-grading raised the wage bill by 4%. Diluting the workforce, on the other hand, reduced wage costs by 12%. The Audit Commission (1992a) and the Clinical Benchmarking Company (CBC 1997) researchers reflected on irrational grading exercises. They noted a 10–30% variation in the number of grade G nurses between districts and in some cases a 20% variation within a district. They concluded that staff mix was irrational rather than logically determined, and recommended that examining the work of all grades of staff was necessary and that opportunities for boosting assistant staff skills through education and training should be taken. These were essential if community services were to expand (Audit Commission 1992a).

Job satisfaction decreased in some areas causing staff to leave. In England generally, posts had been re-graded as vacancies arose. Although some jobs had been upgraded, hours were reduced to keep the exercise cost neutral – little wonder that clinical re-grading was perceived as a cost-cutting exercise. Other downsides included tightly defined job descriptions that limited delegation, which meant that lower-grade nurses refused to act up. Clinical re-grading at least seemed to be at odds with workforce development. In short, few NHS policies have managed to upset both managers and practitioners (Audit Commission 1992a; Gerrish et al. 1998). It is understandable that *Agenda for Change* (DoH 2004) may repeat these mistakes.

# Practice nurses and nurse practitioners

Practice nurses work with GPs and are responsible for implementing prescribed care programmes under the latter's supervision. Nurse practitioners, on the other hand, are usually qualified to at least first-degree level and work alongside their medical colleagues. Although it is important that job titles are not used interchangeably, a more significant difference is that nurse practitioners do not separate task and skill, thereby minimizing the risk of duplication. Nor are they cheaper substitutes for GPs (Rashid et al. 1996; Latimer and Ashburner 1997).

Jeffreys et al. (1995) and Bryar (1994) summarize practice nurses and nurse practitioners' work as:

- preventive
- diagnostic
- patient management, including counselling, health promotion and prescribing.

These chime with the three *Liberating the Talents'* (DoH 2002c) core functions, which recommend ways of advancing the specialist practitioner's role and instigating new primary care services. Practice nurse roles have extended greatly since the job was analysed in detail by the Cumberlege Committee almost 20 years ago. Indeed, 20% of practice nurse and nurse practitioners' work, previously done by GPs, meant that practice nurses may even be changing the nature of GPs' work (Bowling 1985; Jenkins-Clarke and Carr-Hill 1996; Latimer and Ashburner 1997). Health service policy changes have transformed the way primary health-care practitioners are working (Hirst et al. 1998) and the new General Medical Service (GMS) contract (DoH 2002c) is likely to boost practice nurse roles further with both positive and negative consequences (Hyde 2001). For practice nurse and nurse practitioners' roles to develop, several elements have to be in place (DoH 2002c):

- Planning that involves all stakeholders
- Arms' length, supportive managers
- Acknowledging the Nursing and Midwifery Council's (NMC's) professional code of conduct
- Scoping the workforce's knowledge and skills
- Drawing on the latest Department of Health policies
- Working with Workforce Development Confederations (WDCs) to provide education and training
- Developing mentors and supervisors
- Using Changing Workforce programme guidelines
- Setting specific aims and objectives for practitioners
- Measuring the effects of staff-mix changes.

Buckle and Gallen (2003) suggest that *Liberating the Talents'* core functions will boost the number of nurse-led clinics, require a richer grade mix and additional staff to cover time out. Hill and Rutter (2001) and Tudor-Hart (1985a) felt that developing the roles of practice nurses and nurse practitioners can improve access to primary care. Those PCTs that are practice nurse rich (and the range is large) are well placed in this regard, although, as we saw in Chapter 3, the picture is complicated and confused.

Early evidence shows that patients are as satisfied with practice nurses as they are with GP services of the same type. Practice nurses also cover their costs because they generate income for GPs (Jeffreys et al. 1995). Richardson et al. (1998) suggests that 30–32% of GPs could be replaced by other professionals, reducing GP establishments by 32%, and thereby saving £300m (1995 prices). Unsurprisingly, GPs become concerned about their livelihoods and question whether nurses have been educated and trained to the same level as medical practitioners. There are doubts about nurses' confidence and, on the other hand, about over-confident nurses. They are also worried that nurses do not have the same prescribing and certifying powers (discussed earlier). Finally, GPs believe that structural and procedural barriers impede these developments (Rashid et al. 1996; Wilson et al. 2002). Many of these issues can be overcome by raising practitioners' awareness of successes elsewhere. Joint education events, which are now commonplace in PCTs, also help while managers develop more flexible employment arrangements. All these are needed if nurse practitioners are to be accepted (Wilson et al. 2002).

In view of these positive and negative issues, the MPC (2001) and Rashid et al. (1996) raise some interesting questions:

- Do nurses' longer consultation times alter efficiency and effectiveness?
- Is the GP's workload reduced?
- If patients see both GPs and nurse practitioners, is work being duplicated?
- Although patient satisfaction is at least the same, are the public's perceptions altered and risks increased?
- What impact will NHS Direct and walk-in centres have?
- Is resolving the doctor shortage using skill substitution merely passing the problem along?
- Is basic and post-basic education keeping ahead of these changes?
- Do nurses have the same personal liability litigation cover?
- Will nurses accept 24-hour responsibility for patients (although the new GMS contract alters medical practitioners' duties anyway)?

During the author's fieldwork, managers acknowledged that specialist practitioners were not only well trained but also more autonomous and experienced greater job satisfaction. The converse may also be true, i.e. one controversial notion in the literature was that, although some practitioners become advanced, the remainder, as a consequence, became general support staff (Syson-Nibbs 1997). In recognition of this danger the Department of Health (2002c) recommends the following:

- Leadership that supports and encourages flexible working across professional and organizational boundaries
- Letting generalists focus on the community's heath needs
- Working with WDCs to develop comprehensive learning programmes

- Mentoring and supervision
- Integrating workforce planning and development
- Developing self-managed integrated nursing teams
- Delegating and being sensitive to new roles
- Measuring service improvements.

Some of the foregoing affects other professional groups in different ways.

## District nurses

The nature and value of district nurses have been studied extensively, e.g. the Audit Commission (1999) describes a curate's egg. The Commission's researchers accepted that more district nurses would be needed because early discharge patients required more technical care in the community and because of increasing patient expectations. However, the proportion of district nurses in a trust's workforce is double in some PCTs and the time that they spend in direct care can vary as much. The Audit Commission (1999) and McIntosh et al. (2000) felt that at best community nursing grade mix is historical and at worst irrational. Prideaux (1996) classifies district nursing work as:

1. technical, needing qualified nurses
2. basic, no nurse training required
3. ambiguous, could be (1) or (2) depending on the context.

Clearly, (2) would should be jettisoned from district nurses' job description by appropriate staff-mix reviews, whereas (3) might be tolerated by managers and clinicians. As discussed elsewhere, the pressure on district nurses to become leaders, delegators, managers, educators and supervisors is growing. Correcting job dissatisfaction as a consequence of these changes may be achieved by boosting district nurses' advanced practitioner work (DoH 1993b).

## Community staff nurses

Community staff nurses are district nurses without a formal community care qualification. This limits their promotion in the community – a point addressed specifically by the Audit Commission (1999) and the Department of Health (1993b). They are deemed to be ideal primary and community support workers (Syson-Nibbs 1997). If 24-hour and complex care programmes are to be implemented, this particular workforce will need boosting. However, one consequence of community staff nurse growth is that district nurses will increasingly take on leadership, supervision and coordination roles and spend less time in direct patient care. The Audit Commission (1992a) and Evers et al. (1991a, 1991b), on the other hand, explain that basic work need not always be done by lower staff grades. Indeed, job satisfaction and efficiency can be improved by employing higher-grade nurses when, for example, a combination of basic and technical care is needed by the patients, which can be completed, efficiently and effectively, during one district nurse's visit (Cowley 1993).

## Health visitors

Health visitors seem particularly sensitive to the negative implications of staff-mix reviews. As far back as the mid-1980s, Bell and Moules (1985) questioned whether health visitors should be looking after both school-age children and, at the other extreme, elderly patients whereas Gibbing (1995, p. 44) writes:

> Dilution in nursing is nowhere more apparent than in health visiting where nursery nurses, for example, take on health visiting advisory/parenting skills education and development checks. However, saying that it needs a health visitor to carry out certain tasks is hard to argue when the bulk of health care is done by lay-carers . . . fears that skill-mix studies will reduce the demand for highly skilled, higher paid professionals are real. But what's wrong with community nurses acting as a leader and teacher while delegating tasks to formal and informal carers?

Billingham (1991) acknowledges the breadth and depth of health visiting and the issues raised, and suggests three important but competing health visiting roles:

1. Family health specialist, notably health promotion
2. Parental support and child protection
3. Public health worker.

Should the health visitor establishments be increased so that all three domains are adequately covered? If not, then should they specialize and narrow their role? Should other or new roles be developed to replace any jettisoned work? Despite evidence to the contrary (e.g. from health needs analysis), the health visitors' role is falling (DoH 2002c). Wright (1998) recommends, therefore, that health visitors be involved in staff reviews. Indeed, two-thirds of health visitors in Wright's study (1998) said that local staff mix was inappropriate and almost half felt that getting the mix right would help community practitioners to work appropriately, efficiently and effectively (especially clerically and administratively). Importantly, from both a top-down and a bottom-up standpoint, where health visitors have initiated skill-mix reviews, the outcomes have been deemed successful (Buckingham and Wilson 1997).

Health visiting is an expensive service because of their higher grades (Ebeid 2000), so the proportion of health visitors in primary and community teams should be decided by demographic and morbidity as well as financial factors (Gibbing 1995). Increasing patient dependency and high-technology care in the community means that more and more practitioners are specializing. In the case of health visiting, for example, the CBC researchers (1997) and McDonald et al. (1997) noted that trusts were creating specialist health visitors (Table 4.1).

**Table 4.1** Specialist health visitors in different trusts

| Specialist health visitors | Percentage of trusts ($n = 102$) |
| --- | --- |
| Child protection | 60 |
| Special needs | 25 |
| Tuberculosis | 20 |
| Homeless people | 15 |
| Elderly people | 12 |
| Other | 10 |

Possibly as a result of the constant threat hanging over health visitors, there have been moves to create specialist health visitors who work between primary and secondary care, such as breast care and nutritional advice in residential homes (DoH 1993c). Initiatives elsewhere included prevention and promotion specialists such as osteoporosis practitioners who also have an important role liaising with hospital staff to coordinate admission and discharge. Those practitioners focusing on elderly care quickly developed expertise in assessing elderly people's health and social care needs and liaising with statutory and voluntary services. Improvements in efficiency and effectiveness, and especially relief of pressures on hospital services, could be a natural consequence of these developments (Young 1997).

Community care workload issues emerge from new working relationships such as health-visiting assistants. One concern is the amount of time (around 30%) that health visitors spend on administrative and clerical work (Ebeid 2000), which could increase if supervisory work increases. Falling direct care also affects health visitors' relationships with patients and their job satisfaction (Buckingham and Wilson 1997). Nevertheless, health-visiting assistants not only reduced costs but were also judged to be credible and non-threatening. Parents' satisfaction was not diminished because crisis-oriented contacts were replaced by routine visits. Preventive work grew and mothers' well-being improved. GPs seemed more aware of the health visitors' presence. The job satisfaction of health-visiting assistants was high but some were disappointed that their roles could not expand because of a lack of knowledge and skills (Syson-Nibbs 1997).

## School nurses

School nurses promote pupils' health and well-being, which help adolescents to reach their potential. These practitioners assess, diagnose and refer, as well as support, children. Recently Cotton et al. (2000) and the Department of Health (2002b) re-examined the school nurse's role. They concluded that school nurses should be PCT managed, their number and mix empirically determined, and they should work in clusters but aligned to schools. Importantly, new roles are likely to cause school nurses to jettison their substantial screening duties in favour of preventive, diagnostic and treatment work in sexual health, enuresis, bereavement and other contexts. They are also more likely to specialize in asthma care, for example, and to work closely with other agencies (McDonald et al. 1997; DoH 2001b).

However, school-nurse investment varies greatly among PCTs (Cotton et al. 2000). Professional boundaries may be preventing school nurses from expanding their roles, which has been advocated for many years (Bell and Moules 1985; Buckingham and Wilson 1997). Some school nurses felt exploited when health visitor and social carer responsibilities were 'dumped in their laps', which caused Richards et al. (2000) to suggest that a new type of NHS handmaiden was emerging. Syson-Nibbs (1997) felt that school and specialist children's nurses' roles were blurring, conflict was likely and supervision and support during home visits were needed. Nicholson (1998) blames lack of understanding of roles and lack of money to increase the school nursing establishment for these untoward developments.

## Nursery nurses

Clearly, there is a cascade effect when staff mix is reviewed, e.g. Lochead (1994) suggests that nursery nurses could help school nurses to use their special skills. Lochead noted that school nurses were receptive and positive about nursery nurses acting as their assistants, but joint working was not always satisfactory. Assistants were fully occupied and the time released for school nurses was filled by home visits and special clinics. Unfortunately extending assistants' role was hampered by lack of money, equipment and education. Basic training and mentorship are also essential if these changes are to succeed.

Nursery nurses have also been piloted as health-visiting assistants. Their work involved developing parenting skills and health promotion but they were unhappy about immunizing children. Nursery nurses filled vacant health visitor posts, but more were needed to achieve the same outputs and outcomes as health visitors. Therefore, the pilot programme did not save money. On the other hand, one effect of the change was to release health visitors for more public health work (Seymour 1994).

# Health-care assistants

As raised earlier, health-care assistants have an important and growing role in primary and community care, which ranges from clinic duties to work in the patient's home (Audit Commission 1994; Ebeid 2000). Richards et al. (2000) argued that 30% of nurses' work could be delegated to assistants, making them a valuable and a better-used member of the primary health-care team. Time saved by delegating administrative work alone was the equivalent of at least 2.5 hours each week. Clearly, health-care assistants make substantial personal, technical and administrative contributions that reduce inappropriate working among qualified nurses, thereby improving efficiency and effectiveness (Hirst et al. 1998; DoH 2002b).

Meadows et al. (2000) indicated that the proportion of health-care assistants in the workforce has remained constant at around 25%, which partly allays fears and refutes the argument that the workforce is being diluted for financial reasons. However, the proportion of nursing assistants in PCTs varies widely, with no obvious rationale except that community staffing tends to be historical (Table 4.2).

**Table 4.2** District nurses and health-care assistants (HCAs) per capita

| PCT/Band | HCAs | District nurses |
|---|---|---|
| England | 1:3986 | 1:5059 |
| Three-star PCTs | 4129 | 5131 |
| ONS Band 1 PCTs | 4055 | 5632 |
| ONS Band 2 | 5124 | 4573 |
| ONS Band 3 | 5428 | 6886 |
| ONS Band 4 | 3006 | 5324 |
| ONS Band 5 | 3960 | 5078 |
| ONS Band 6 | 3240 | 4901 |
| Specimen Band 3 PCT | 7101 | 4890 |
| Specimen's percentile | 75th | 45th |

Kendall and Lissauer (2003) reminded us that 144 000 extra assistants are needed (throughout the NHS) if nurses are to extend their roles. McDonald et al. (1997), Buchan (1998) and Buchan and Edwards (2000), on the other hand, warn that increasing numbers of health-care assistants should be carefully monitored because of reasons raised earlier, such as the effect on qualified staff's work patterns. The danger of shifting qualified staff from practitioner to supervisor roles has consequences not only for outputs and outcomes but also for job satisfaction, recruitment and retention.

One-third of general practices employ practice nurse assistants, so healthcare assistants, similar to their registered practitioner counterparts, are specializing. Practice nursing is one discipline that is likely to depend on health-care assistants in the future because of the 'greying' practice nurse workforce (Wright 2002), discussed in Chapter 7.

The morbidity and socioeconomic data discussed in Chapter 3 offer plenty of scope for health promotion and disease prevention. For health-care assistants to play a vital role, they will need greater knowledge and skills if these kinds of duties increase in the community. Assistants who specialize may need educating and training to level 3 NVQ (National Vocational Qualification) and even then registered nurses should delegate only those tasks that assistants are capable of doing and carefully supervise their work (McDonald et al. 1997; Elkan et al. 2000; McIntosh et al. 2000; Richards et al. 2000). Also, patients need to understand the difference between registered and unregistered staff, and risk assessments ought to include health-care assistants' work. Feelings about these developments are mixed and are similar to staff-mix reservations discussed elsewhere. Some GPs support practice nurse assistants, whereas elsewhere both GPs and practice nurses feared that roles were being usurped and the profession destabilized (Rapport and Maggs 1997; Royal College of Nursing or RCN 1997; Wright 2002). Even careful supervision and extra education, will not prepare nursing assistants to replace qualified nurses fully so these fears are likely to disappear.

Analysing health-visiting assistants' activity is illuminating even though the data are old. Commonly, their time was spent guiding, advising and helping older patients with:

- aids and appliances
- medication
- financial issues
- mobility
- nutrition
- carer relief.

Encouragingly, care was based on patient assessments so, theoretically, the most dependent patients attracted the most attention. Continuity was strong because a small number of patients accounted for most activities (Williams et al. 1992). Cochrane et al. (2002), as part of the Future Healthcare Workforce (FHCW) programme, set out a job description for the older person's practitioner assistant role, which included assessment, investigation, diagnosis, treatment and care.

# Paraprofessionals

Elkan et al. (2000a, 2000b, 2000c) noted that paraprofessionals attracted interest in the international and local literature. Homestart and Newpin used parent volunteers to support parents but the practice did not become widely accepted or adopted in the UK (Audit Commission 1994). However, these paraprofessionals were good at helping families in deprived areas, running family clinics and giving support in the parent's home. Although no studies have formally compared paraprofessional efficiency and effectiveness, perceptions were that professionals were released for more pressing work. Paraprofessionals may be more accepted culturally and obviously are cheaper. However, they should not work alone or unsupervised and are likely to need continuing support from professionals. Also, managers should be aware that any gaps between professional and paraprofessional roles allow vulnerable parents and children to slip through the net. Child abuse is deemed to be one danger area and complex cases such as these should not be delegated. There is also a worry that these workers become a cadre of unpaid (or low paid at best) workers which further demeans and devalues women's work (Elkan et al. 2000a, 2000b, 2000c).

# Allied health professionals

Probably because allied health professionals (AHPs) can be employed by session in general practices, the number and, more so, the mix of substantive AHPs' WTE (whole-time equivalent) posts in PCTs varies irrationally (Table 4.3).

**Table 4.3** Allied health professionals per capita

| PCT/Band | Podiatrists | Dietitians | Occupational therapists | Physio- therapists | Speech and language therapists |
|---|---|---|---|---|---|
| England | 1:13 466 | 1:31 927 | 1:12 166 | 1:9485 | 1:9609 |
| Three-star PCTs | 11 401 | 22 210 | 8377 | 7687 | 10 911 |
| ONS Band 1 PCTs | 14 931 | 92 445 | 15 242 | 21 323 | 10 253 |
| ONS Band 2 | 10 494 | 17 655 | 14 597 | 8876 | 9743 |
| ONS Band 3 | 14 159 | 41 352 | 25 089 | 15 929 | 9272 |
| ONS Band 4 | 14 030 | 26 769 | 10 050 | 8309 | 9560 |
| ONS Band 5 | 14 999 | 32 518 | 13 586 | 8587 | 9148 |
| ONS Band 6 | 13 473 | 31 154 | 9109 | 8725 | 11 479 |
| Specimen Band 3 PCT | NA* | 60 268 | 26 698 | 10 679 | NA |
| Specimen's percentile | | 75th | 75th | 57th | |

*NA, not employed.

Some health-care professionals, particularly AHPs, are in a seller's market and have the upper hand. They are at the top of the low unemployment league. Although this gives practitioners an edge, one consequence is a further dilution of the health-care workforce as trusts struggle to recruit qualified staff in favour of health-care assistants (Buchan 1998; Buchan and Edwards 2000). These issues are discussed further in Chapter 7. Fieldwork by the author showed that graduates from courses not usually associated with clinical practice were being employed as nutritionists to help ease the increasing dietetic workload caused by unfilled vacancies. However, one manager felt that she was at a saturation point with assistant grades. She was worried that professional involvement in direct care would continue to fall as a consequence of qualified staff supervising more assistant grades (discussed earlier in other contexts). Other managers were conscious of extended roles. One podiatrist, for example, said that orthopaedic patient fast tracking, which placed the bulk of care on to podiatrists, not only made patient care more efficient but also raised practitioners' job satisfaction. Moreover, boosting podiatrist curative roles is cost-efficient and effective.

## Administrative and clerical staff

Support staff are rarely included in staff reviews despite the effect they have on efficiency and effectiveness (Rodriguez 1994). Consequently, their connection to GPs and practice nurses is important (Table 4.4).

**Table 4.4** GPs, practice nurses and administrative staff per capita

| PCT/Band | GPs (list size) | Practice nurses | Administrative staff |
|---|---|---|---|
| England | 1:2009 | 1:4582 | 1:999 |
| Three-star PCTs | 1932 | 4509 | 989 |
| ONS Band 1 PCTs | 2136 | 4889 | 984 |
| ONS Band 2 | 1981 | 4467 | 928 |
| ONS Band 3 | 2015 | 4375 | 987 |
| ONS Band 4 | 2040 | 4845 | 1019 |
| ONS Band 5 | 1968 | 4797 | 1046 |
| ONS Band 6 | 1954 | 4437 | 999 |
| Specimen Band 3 PCT | 2033 | 3556 | 924 |
| Specimen's percentile | 65th | 6th | 21st |

Our case study PCT is practice administrative and clerical staff rich. There may be scope, therefore, for delegating community practitioners' administrative and clerical work to practice clerical staff. However, as the Medical Practices Committee (MPC 2001) points out, evidence supporting this move is thin.

## Managers

Similar to administrative and clerical staff, first-line, middle and senior manager staff-mix implications are not always considered. No empirically determined evidence about the implications of staff changes for managers could be located in the literature. Nevertheless, the Audit Commission (1992a) reminded readers that numbers and types of managers need to change in line with the broader picture. Changes, however, should not leave the service under-managed. Tangentially, a comparison between managers' and practitioners' views of primary and community care offers interesting insights into workforce planning and development (Rapport and Maggs 1997) (Table 4.5).

**Table 4.5** Views of managers and practitioners

| Managers' views | Practitioners' views |
| --- | --- |
| Managers understand patients and their needs | Managers are too remote and out of touch |
| There are plenty of opportunities for practitioners to update themselves | Managers offered too few opportunities for funded study leave |
| Managers are left out of the primary and community care policy reforms | Gap between managers and practitioners has widened and there is little shared vision |
| Practitioners were accountable for direct patient care | Managers unaware of the additional work elements and pressures facing practitioners |

Although these perceptions are only indirectly related to workforce planning and development, they have bearing on the professional judgement approach to the size and mix of health-care teams (see Chapter 8). Trust staff mix by the various PCT groupings explored is shown in Table 4.6 (overleaf).

Apart from one or two staff groups, PCT staff mix is remarkably uniform, which questions the claim that PCT workforce planning is irrational.

Table 4.6 Staff mix

| PCT/Band | HVs (%) | DNs (%) | SNs (%) | HCAs (%) | GPs (%) | PNs (%) | Admin staff (%) | Podiatrists (%) | Dietitians (%) | OTs (%) | PTs (%) | SaLTs (%) |
|---|---|---|---|---|---|---|---|---|---|---|---|---|
| Three-star PCTs | 5.2 | 5.6 | 10.3 | 9.2 | 17.9 | 6.7 | 30.1 | 2.7 | 1.2 | 3.5 | 3.7 | 3.8 |
| ONS Band 1 PCTs | 6.4 | 5.7 | 12.5 | 7.9 | 19.1 | 6.6 | 32.6 | 2.2 | 0.3 | 2.1 | 1.5 | 3.1 |
| ONS Band 2 | 6.4 | 6.6 | 13 | 5.9 | 15.4 | 6.8 | 32.7 | 2.9 | 1.7 | 1.3 | 3.4 | 3.1 |
| ONS Band 3 | 6.3 | 4.8 | 13.9 | 6.1 | 18 | 7.5 | 33.3 | 2.3 | 0.8 | 3.1 | 2.1 | 3.6 |
| ONS Band 4 | 5.5 | 5.8 | 9.8 | 10.3 | 18.2 | 6.4 | 30.5 | 2.2 | 1.2 | 2.4 | 3.7 | 3.3 |
| ONS Band 5 | 6.1 | 6.5 | 8.2 | 8.3 | 19.3 | 6.9 | 31.6 | 2.2 | 1 | 3.3 | 3.8 | 3.6 |
| ONS Band 6 | 5.7 | 6.2 | 10.3 | 9.4 | 18.2 | 6.9 | 30.5 | 2.3 | 1 | 0.1 | 3.5 | 2.7 |
| Specimen Band 3 PCT | 7.4 | 5.8 | 28.2 | 4 | 15.4 | 7.9 | 24.8 | 0 | 0.5 | 8.6 | 0.3 | 0 |

PCT, primary care trust; HVs, health visitors; DNs, district nurses; SNs, community staff nurses; HCAs, health-care assistants; OTs, occupational therapists; PTs, physiotherapists; SaLTs, speech and language therapists.

## Multidisciplinary and integrated teams

The Department of Health (1993a) noted more than a decade ago that stronger working relationships between a wide range of statutory and voluntary services suggest that integration is possible. Multidisciplinary and integrated teams bring staff mix sharply into focus. Latimer and Ashburner (1997) felt that it is increasingly difficult for individuals and even individual professional groups to justify their contributions and one solution is to think about the workforce as a homogeneous group.

Researchers find little relationship between primary health-care team structure and mode of working. Delegation and referral, for example, seem no more rational in multidisciplinary settings than elsewhere (Editorial 1997). *Making a Difference* (DoH 1999a) recommended that primary health-care teams work together for effectiveness and efficiency. Consequently, integrated working has become an important aim in view of demand and supply variables influencing different professional groups (Buchan and Edwards 2000; DoH 2001b). Moreover, NSFs encourage multidisciplinary working (DoH 2002g), e.g. the Diabetes and the Older Person's NSFs raised two issues:

1. having sufficient staff to meet service demands
2. developing a workforce that achieves high-quality care.

The GP shortfall, particularly in the case study PCT, could jeopardize these plans without at least maintaining or boosting the nursing and AHP workforces (DoH 2002e).

The way chronic diseases are being managed by health and social care professionals working in different organizations in the same locality also calls for integrated workforce planning and development (Hyde 2001; Kendall and Lissauer 2003). Initial workforce planning actions include agreeing respective roles with other agencies and capitalizing by harmonizing health and social care needs' assessment (Constantinides and Gorden 1990; Lightfoot 1993). Moving from hierarchically arranged community structures to integrated teams:

- generates opportunities for more efficient and effective working
- capitalizes on a growing trend towards multidisciplinary primary and community teams
- improves the continuity and coordination of care
- reduces duplication
- makes better use of skills
- improves job satisfaction
- strengthens peer learning
- improves the opportunity to share protocols
- dilutes the reliance on one staff group.

Unfortunately, there are downsides (Cartlidge et al. 1987b; Wiles and Robinson 1994; Hodder 1995; Poulton 1996; CBC 1997; Latimer and Ashburner 1997; McDonald et al. 1997; Rapport and Maggs 1997; Bull 1998; Holland 1998; Audit Commission 1999; Buchan and Edwards 2000; Hyde 2001; DoH 2002b; Kendall and Lissauer 2003):

- Integrated team leaders with no greater recognition or reward for their extra responsibility
- Heightened anxieties, jealousies and unclear boundaries that mar working relationships
- Uneven commitment in localities
- Teams not being centrally based
- Lacking evidence that integrated teams improve the quality of care
- Falling direct care and rising administrative and clerical work
- Inequitable study leave and budgets, and inappropriate use of staff at the time of shortages such as weekends and holidays
- Staff in the lower echelons feeling ignored or put upon
- Varying employment and contracting conditions encouraging territorialism, protectionism and fragmentation which lead at least to communication difficulties
- Common learning programmes years down the line.

Cartlidge et al. (1987b), Rapport and Maggs (1997) and Wiles and Robinson (1994) measured several teamwork issues and some results were surprisingly poor. Outcomes varied between professionals – health visitors and midwives were particularly dissatisfied with teamwork whereas social workers felt that barriers between services led to problems.

Following on from the first point immediately above, there is a debate in the literature about who leads integrated teams. The Audit Commission (1994) felt that health visitors were well placed to coordinate and develop child health and Social Services, whereas Wiles and Robinson's (1994) study showed that GPs were natural leaders as a result of their legal responsibility for patients. Despite this obvious fact, there is a view among some staff that medical practitioners became leaders because of their power and status in the NHS. PMS projects, on the other hand, were reversing the legal responsibility, power and status issues (Kendall and Lissauer 2003).

Health-care and social care-integrated working problems may need different solutions, although new policy initiatives ought to be tried and evaluated. There is an inevitability about these developments as new workers, who cut across health and social care boundaries, emerge, especially among the non-registered workforce. A new, unexpected problem seems to be emerging for district nurses who have seen varying amounts of work shift to Social Services. This demarcation is undermining the district nurse's role as aspects of patients' care fall beyond the social care workers' abilities, which once again becomes the NHS workers' responsibility. In some cases, district nurs-es became out of touch with the patients' health-care and social care needs (Hesketh 2002).

## The Changing Workforce and Future Healthcare Workforce programmes

One clear message in the most recent workforce planning and development literature is that 'more of the same' model is no longer an option (Andrews 2004). It was inevitable, therefore, that the FHCW project focused on pri-mary and community care (Cochrane et al. 2002). The effects of the NSFs and modernization programmes, which call for new ways of doing things if targets and standards are to be met, are already being felt. The Changing Workforce Programme (CWP) (DoH 2001b) and the FHCW report encour-age innovative working. They were established to support front-line staff and improve patient services by making better use of staff skills. It is anticipated that workforce modernization along CWP and FHCW lines could solve recruitment and retention problems.

Role changes are achieved by moving tasks up or down the traditional job ladder. Expanding the breadth and depth of a smaller number of health-care roles should be possible by combining roles and asking the jobholder to work differently. Some practitioners, notably GPs with special interests (GPSIs), are specializing (Obeid 1997; Cochrane et al. 2002; NHS Workforce Taskforce et al. 2002). In short, three staff groups are emerging from these recent developments:

1. Specialists, including consultants, GPs, specialist registrars and clinical specialists (it is not clear why consultant nurses and therapists are not included).
2. Health-care practitioners who combine junior doctor, nursing and thera-py knowledge and skills.
3. Health-care practitioner assistants who incorporate the roles of nursing, therapy and other assistants in the health services and Social Services.

These new practitioners replace existing staff groups. They deliver holis-tic services – ranging from assessment to treatment, care and rehabilitation. Assistants, the patient's main contact, play an important role implementing care plans/protocols/pathways (Kendall and Lissauer 2003). These authors go on to set out the objectives for this modernized workforce:

- Improve relationships between managers and clinicians: equalizing power and control.

- Engendering shared professionalism: closer working between practitioners and sectors.
- Transforming practitioner–patient relationships: a consumerist approach.
- Shifting the dominant medical model towards a psychosocial one.

The relationship between district nursing and social care work is often raised in the context of CWP and FHCW. Latimer and Ashburner (1997), for example, question whether older community patients need the services of qualified nurses. There is a feeling that personal care is the responsibility of Social Services, who support family carers. Cynical writers said that social carers were interested only in forming relationships with health service staff so that some of their overwhelming Social Service caseloads could be passed back to health service staff (McDonald et al. 1997). Whether community practitioners should be delivering social care has been firmly decided in the literature, although there are grey areas where it is hard to draw a line. Although data are old, Evers et al. (1991a, 1991b) looked at the differences between health care and social care, and coined the term 'extra care' to distinguish between community health care and social care. Extra care is defined as social care that needs health-care professionals' contribution such as special diets. Evers et al. (1991a, 1991b) noted several different extra care activities, which suggests that the issue is real rather than imagined.

The Audit Commission (1992a) estimated that 8% of people aged over 65 (0.5% of the total population) were receiving care from health services and Social Services. Managers, during interviews, said that, despite the benefits of interdisciplinary working, boundaries between health and social carers were preventing service developments (Cochrane et al. 2002). Consequently, the CWP Toolkit, backed by the single assessment process, envisaged a new generic worker spanning health and social care sectors. Cochrane et al. (2002), as raised earlier, as part of the FHCW programme, set out a job description for the older person's practitioner which ranged over assessment, investigation, diagnosis, treatment, care and rehabilitation.

Evidence-based protocols are a strong feature of CWP and FHCW, which allow workers to cross the traditional professional boundaries, and enhance career opportunities and job satisfaction. These specify the roles, responsibilities and sequence of interventions for health-care and social care professionals, especially for those who combine both roles (Kendall and Lissauer 2003). There are conflicting views, barriers and difficulties, however. Kendall and Lissauer (2003), for example, make a strong case for specialist health-care workers, not least for reasons of efficiency and effectiveness. These arguments counter those advocating generic working, which may explain why CWP and FHCW progress has been slower than expected. Inevitably, managers questioned whether there has been sufficient investment in modernizing the workforce, although the blame cannot be laid entirely at the Exchequer's door. Not only is there resistance in the workforce (as with staff-mix changes generally) and maintaining professional interests and identities, but also there are doubts about CWP's coherence. These restrictive practices and entrenched values work against workforce modernization. On the one hand, progressive workforce planners have not always engaged health-care professionals who felt on the periphery, which contrasts markedly with their coalface responsibilities, knowledge and experience (Cochrane et al. 2002; Kendall and Lissauer 2003).

Basic and post-basic curricula need major reform if CWP and FHCW plans are to succeed (Hyde 2001; Kendall and Lissauer 2003). The former nursing regulatory body, the UK Central Council (UKCC), considered scrapping separate district nursing and health-visiting qualifications in favour of a combined role such as Ireland's public health nurse (Atkin et al. 1994). Later, this new worker was labelled the 'family health nurse', a generic, multiskilled worker at the centre of primary care. However, there is concern that relatively new roles such as nurse practitioners could be usurped while yet another tier is added to the job ladder (Hyde 2001). Finally, generic working is sensitive as a result of pay differences between health-care and social care staff (DoH 2000a). Clearly, the dividing line between health care and social care is unclear and uncertain. However, it is likely to be increasingly necessary as the numbers of elderly patients cared for at home increase (Betts 2003).

Professional organizations, trade unions and government all agree that changes to working practices are crucial. Yet there is little agreement about the actual shape of the future health-care and social care workforce. Reforms to date have tended to focus on short-term goals such as adjusting staffing so that access to services is improved (Obeid 1997; Kendall and Lissauer 2003). Possibly as a result of recent reorganizations, the regulatory bodies, which remain as compartmentalized as the traditional jobs themselves, have not addressed how the emerging hybrid roles will be registered and monitored, and are seen as another barrier to workforce re-design. Similarly, re-training existing staff is a difficult problem. Preparation and use of competencies to re-design and monitor roles have not been addressed empirically by the statutory bodies, despite being a potential solution (Cochrane et al. 2002; NHS Workforce Taskforce 2002). However, the Skills for Health Team, emerging at the time this book was being written, is addressing competency issues.

Too many practitioners fail to share information and decision-making among themselves and with the patient. One recent policy initiative designed to overcome this problem, and one that is likely to override other staff-mix initiatives, is *Liberating the Talents* (DoH 2002c). The nature and purpose of this initiative are similar to those of CWP and FHCW – streamlining the plethora of primary and community care jobs (Healy 2002a, 2002b). Three core functions have been designed (and described earlier). These new roles were explored extensively in Chapter 3, but the staff-mix issues are reiterated here.

First Contact is likely to be the domain of primary care practitioners, emergency services and walk-in centres, etc. (Harrogate Centre for Excellence in Health and Social Care or HCEHSC 2003). One way of not overburdening these practitioners is by extending health-care assistants' roles so that they can support First Contact workers (Kendall and Lissauer 2003).

Prompted by *Liberating the Talents*' CDM core function, progressive workforce planners have initiated new roles such as the diabetes generic worker, whose role includes education and technical duties. These practitioners undergo additional education and training before they intensively manage patients with diabetes who are poorly controlled or failing to conform. As the efficiency and effectiveness of diabetic care have been greatly improved, new roles for other CDM categories are likely to follow (Healy 2002a, 2002b; Lewis 2003a; Lewis and Rosen 2003).

Despite the importance of disease prevention and health promotion, public health has a chequered history in the NHS. One reason for creating the public health nursing role is that GPs lack the time and in some cases the skills to carry out public health work. Moreover, many GPs consider public health to be a low-status activity and limit their involvement by delegating public health work to nurses. Another long-standing problem is that key public health workers, such as health visitors and school nurses, are employed outside general practices and public health departments, which separates public health science and public health practice. A more straightforward reason why work in this important field has faltered is simply staff shortages (Kendall and Lissauer 2003).

## Conclusion

Despite their different meanings, skill mix (interprofessional) and grade mix (intraprofessional) are often used synonymously in the literature. However, the universal phrase 'staff mix' may be more appropriate and may be more acceptable because its connotations are less negative. Nevertheless, staff mix is an important workforce planning and development issue, not least for cost and quality reasons. There is growing evidence in the literature that achieving the right staffing balance:

- frees skilled professionals from inappropriate duties
- creates a flexible workforce able to work in a more interdisciplinary way
- improves health-care efficiency and effectiveness
- generates good evidence for change if a robust evaluation of change is made
- demands good management and leadership to overcome the sensitivities surrounding an emotive topic
- can ease recruitment and retention difficulties.

With more than a million NHS staff and the myriad of job titles in which they fall, there ought to be scope for streamlining the PCT workforce. However, there is a bewildering array of variables that managers need to consider. Determination of the right staff mix requires complex decisions and even then there is no guarantee that the appropriate mix leads to better services. Evidence about the effect dilute staff mix has on the cost and quality of care, for example, is conflicting in the literature. Fortunately, recent policy and related documents are clear about what staff-mix changes are needed and there are several models such as *Liberating the Talents*, *Making a Difference* (DoH 1999a), Evercare and Kaiser Permanente. These can help managers modernize the workforce, but no model is free of criticism.

Traditional staff-mix decisions are irrational and not always based on sound evidence. Consequently, practitioners may be working less efficiently and effectively, e.g. despite many PCTs having generous administrative staffing, rising levels of clerical and administrative work among clinical staff are an intractable problem. Staff-mix adjustments can be a highly sensitive issue. Managers and clinicians find themselves entrenched and polarized especially when evidence for change is lacking. Despite two-thirds of staff in one survey feeling that the staff mix was wrong, resistance, as a result of anxiety, professional boundaries and jealousies, was a strong restraining force for change. These might be the reasons why NHS staff-mix reviews have a chequered history. Traditional workforce reviews have faltered because the process has not been inclusive or staff-mix recommendations lacked evidence. However, empirical studies indicate that health-care professionals are 'coming round' to fairly and robustly conducted staff-mix reviews. Moving beyond a narrow, cost-cutting agenda and exploring the potential benefit to patients are the main reasons for the increasingly positive perceptions. However, modern primary and community care workforces based on patient needs and shared working will rely on staff understanding modernized workforce planning.

The ratio of qualified to assistant nurses in primary and community care settings varies remarkably and irrationally. Worries about diluting the registered workforce overwhelm those who support boosting the number of health-care assistants. Staff-mix adjustments based on delegation and skill substitution are efficient but may not be effective. As a result of isolated and autonomous work, separation of task and skill in primary and community care may not be wise, particularly for practitioners used to assessing patients, and planning, delivering and evaluating care holistically. Nevertheless, there is mounting evidence that health-care assistants raise both service efficiency and effectiveness. The staff-mix issues facing different professional groups are considerable and for some groups unique.

A review of the literature and analysis of the PCT WP&D database show the following:

- Practice nurses, generalist and specialist nurse practitioners will be strongly influenced by first contact and CDM service developments.
- District nurses, community staff nurses, Social Service carers and healthcare assistants need careful balancing if duplication and reduced service quality are to be avoided.
- The numbers and education of community staff nurses are important if CDM and out-of-hours services are to succeed.
- Health visitors are emerging as the main public health workforce, which may remove once and for all questions about the nature and value of their role. The public health role of school nurses is also strengthening, particularly dealing with teenage health issues.
- Other health workers such as nursery nurses and paraprofessionals are attracting managers' attention, especially their health-visiting and school nurse assistant roles.
- The proportion of health-care assistants, despite sound evidence about their value to PCT members, is double in some PCTs. However, their numbers although irrational are historical rather than cost driven.
- Similarly, the proportion of AHPs in the PCT workforce fluctuates and seems equally irrational. Interestingly, three-star PCTs have proportionally more AHPs in their workforce.

The volume and complexity of health and social care needed in the home, health centre and other community settings are likely to change in the near future. Any response from PCT managers has to be patient and community centred, multidisciplinary, multiagency, flexible and creative. The long-standing NHS specialist–generalist debate is unlikely to settle, but there is evidence that shifting complex care into the hands of a smaller number of specialist practitioners is likely to improve efficiency and effectiveness. Expecting generalists, on the other hand, to deal with the remaining mundane work is not only unfair but also has job satisfaction, recruitment and retention implications. However, this is an over-simplification. Patient-focused, interdisciplinary and integrated workforce planning will steadily replace uniprofessional approaches as a result of the growing number of interrelated variables such as *Liberating the Talents*, NSFs and supply-side problems. Although staff-mix reviews for a modernized NHS are well argued theoretically, data and algorithms are thin on the ground. Consequently, professional judgement has to be used to adjust staff mix in these situations. Nevertheless, the FHCW programme and CWP are increasingly influencing primary and community health-care teams, which offer useful guidance for managers. Innovative jobs are emerging but progress is hampered because education and professional regulation are lagging.

The challenge facing managers is to respond to patients' needs while at the same time accepting that resources are limited. Consequently, managers realize that staff-mix reviews should not be taken lightly. Indeed, independent authors suggest that a staff-mix code of practice and protocol are needed. In short, for staff-mix changes to succeed PCT managers need to consider population size, health needs' assessment such as disability, financial constraints, local and national policies, etc., as well as being sensitive to professionals' feelings about role changes. Evaluation and adjustment of staff mix can be made easier if the issues affecting specific staff groups are considered and guidance comes from two sources:

1. systematic reviews of the literature that give a national overview of staff mix
2. Office for National Statistics/Department of Health databases that provide data and benchmarks.

Items 1 and 2 are explored in more detail later.

# CHAPTER FIVE

# Efficiency and effectiveness

## Introduction and background

Lewis and deBene (1994) suggested that the move from secondary to primary care has inherent benefits, e.g. social dislocation is reduced and patient satisfaction increases whereas appropriate staffing improves service efficiency and effectiveness. Quality and cost of primary and community care, an alternative heading to efficiency and effectiveness in a workforce-planning context, are linked theoretically and practically, e.g. one primary care trust (PCT) studied by the author, although highly productive and efficiently staffed, had the second highest reference cost (average cost per community care episode) of all PCTs (Table 5.1).

**Table 5.1** Reference costs

| PCT/Band | Index |
| --- | --- |
| England | 113 |
| Three-star PCTs | 102 |
| ONS Band 1 PCTs | 147 |
| ONS Band 2 | 101 |
| ONS Band 3 | 114 |
| ONS Band 4 | 112 |
| ONS Band 5 | 123 |
| ONS Band 6 | 109 |
| Specimen Band 3 PCT | 171 |
| Specimen's percentile | 88th |

Reference costs can be thought of as the figure above or below the average cost per case, e.g. our specimen PCT in Table 5.1 has an average cost per case that is 71% above the average (taken as 100). There are many PCTs that exceed the average level and it is likely that staff costs contribute significantly to reference costs. Indeed, the majority of the NHS bill is accounted for by wages and community nurses explain a third of the primary and community care wages bill. Adjusting the size and mix of community teams can change the wages bill anywhere from –8% to +4%. Quality and costs are, therefore, inseparable when planning and developing the workforce (Audit Commission 1992a). In view of managers' increasing scrutiny of health-care costs it has never been more important for community practitioners to demonstrate their worth as professionals compete for resources. Undoubtedly, workforce planning and development are connected to service efficiency and effectiveness, which can be enhanced using local and national data.

# Workforce planning, development and quality from a methodological perspective

Both the government's and the public's expectations for the quality of health-care services are rising (Piggott 1988). Consequently, practitioners are expected to measure outcomes to demonstrate the value of their services. Moreover, clinical governance made service quality improvement a statutory duty for all NHS trusts, which may explain why quality became a formal requirement of the new General Medical Services (GMS) contract. Trust managers will be expected to demonstrate not only the range of their primary and community care services but also their effect (Proctor and Campbell 1999; Fatchett and Gleeson 2002; NHS Workforce Taskforce et al. 2002). Toms (1992, p. 1489) defines community quality as:

> the overall experience and satisfaction of the patient with . . . service from [referral] to discharge.

Recent Department of Health policy, notably the National Service Frameworks (NSFs), places quality of care at its heart, especially the reduction of unacceptable service variations. Implicitly, primary and community care should meet not only 'equity' but also the other five Maxwellian dimensions of quality, which potentially saves the NHS money (Proctor and Campbell 1999; DoH 2002g).

### Maxwell's quality dimensions

1. Effectiveness of services: doing the right things. These can be measured by clinical governance system checks such as the evidence basis of pathways/protocols.
2. Efficiency and economy: doing things right, measured, for example, using generic prescribing or comparing services against targets.
3. Equity or fair service distribution: measured by the relationship between health needs analysis and resources.

4. Access to services not limited by time and place: usually measured by auditing clinic opening times, home visits and triage systems.
5. Acceptability of services that meets patients' wants and needs: indicated by patient satisfaction measures.
6. Relevance of service to patients' wants and needs: sometimes measured using health gain indicators.

Proctor and Campbell (1999) welcome the move away from efficiency measures to a fuller consideration of Maxwell's dimensions. However, measuring all six dimensions is not easy and it is unlikely that the decisions about which performance indicators to use will be reached by consensus. Another challenge facing workforce planners and developers, as Toms (1992) noted, is that quality improvement programmes may have little influence on service quality. Consequently, managers will find it difficult to attribute good or poor performance to staffing changes.

Nevertheless, clinical governance requirements mean that managers have to make progress. Rowe and Mackeith (1991) summarize community quality measures in three ways:

1. Patient-completed questionnaires about, for example, first contact and follow-up.
2. Group measures that plot patients' progress against agreed targets.
3. Peer review: staff compare themselves against best practice.

From the author's review the most popular community quality improvement methods in the literature were the following (Waite 1986; Anderson 1991; Rink et al. 1996; Clinical Benchmarking Company or CBC 1997; West and Poulton 1997; Audit Commission 1999; Almond 2002; DoH 2002d; Stevenson et al. 2003):

- Quality standards
- Patient and staff satisfaction surveys
- Quality pointer-type judgements on the adequacy and safety of home visits in the context of workload
- Outcome and output data monitoring
- Performance indicators, such as prescribing rates
- Mortality and morbidity data
- Activity analysis such as practitioner–patient interaction
- Performance appraisal
- Care pathway variance analyses
- Benchmarking
- Proxy measures of quality such as leg ulcer treatment, incontinence management and general assessment processes.

Not only is the list incomplete but also each approach has strengths and weaknesses, and none is free of criticism, e.g. structures and process measures predominate, a point also noted by the Audit Commission (1992a). Rowe and Mackeith (1991) believe that some outcome/output indicators (such as immunization rates) are too simplistic and offer perverse incentives because one service is boosted to meet targets at the expense of others. However, Proctor and Campbell (1999) confirm that primary and community care outcomes are hard to agree and even more difficult to measure owing to the socioeconomic influences on clinical outcomes and the range of stakeholders involved.

Clearly, the Healthcare Commission (2003 – see http://ratings2004. healthcarecommission.org.uk/Trust/Overview/mht_overview.asp) star ratings have boosted health-care outcome and output measurement from the low number of primary and community care outcomes gathered by the Department of Health and Office of National Statistics (ONS) (Audit Commission 1992a). The methods used in a workforce planning and development context fall neatly into categories.

## Standard-setting methods

Community standards (the first in the list of commonly used methods) have a chequered history. Constructing standards using consensus has been difficult and sometimes they have been extrapolated without testing their psychometric properties. Consequently, autonomous and remote working in the community may mean that auditors encounter varying practices or that measures are less valid and reliable. Of the commercially available ones, Monitor (Illsley and Goldstone 1987) is the best known but the 'package' is relatively expensive and has been accused of generating snapshots only. Monitor is nursing structure and process oriented, which at least makes it patient centred (Illsley and Goldstone 1986; Toms 1992; Poulton and West 1994). An alternative and comprehensive source of community standards is the Trent Package. This includes statements, audit questions and interpretation guidance that overcome Monitor's outcome weaknesses by tracking the community patient from referral to discharge (Trent Health 1991).

Phillip et al. (1990) describe a North American system used for care of elderly people based on non-participation observation in the patients' homes, which includes six quality-of-care dimensions:

1. physical
2. medical
3. management and financial
4. psychosocial
5. environmental
6. human rights.

These six dimensions include 53 standards and measuring criteria scored from best to worst possible care. Encouragingly, the instrument's psychometric properties are well tested and appear sound.

*The Essence of Care* (DoH 2002d), a benchmarking system, is attracting attention in the UK and may correct the structure, process and outcome imbalance of current measures. This document is designed to improve care quality by systematically comparing good and poor practice and remedying weaknesses. Data are qualitative, although empirically derived numerical indicators are emerging:

- Self-care
- Food and nutrition
- Hygiene
- Elimination
- Pressure sores
- Record keeping
- Privacy and dignity
- Safety.

For each element there is/are:

- an overall statement of what is expected
- indicators that range from worst to best practice (as in Phillip et al. 1990)
- ways of highlighting practices that need attention
- patient expectations
- information sources
- a scoring sheet
- an action plan.

## Document analysis

Nursing records-based quality assurance, although valuable, raises important methodological issues, e.g. auditor access to patient-held records is not easy and document design and language may not be standard, which may limit comparisons and benchmarking. Practitioners may be suspicious about auditors' backgrounds, i.e. managers have different perspectives to clinicians because the former are budget oriented. Also from the practitioner's standpoint, neither peer review nor self-audit is liked as a result of the administrative burden. Finally, document reviews are usually based on short-term care episodes and may not have the continuity element of the inpatient counterpart (Illsley and Goldstone 1986; Toms 1992). Despite these limitations the Audit Commission (1999) showed the value of document reviews:

1. 53% (SD = 20%) of the general assessments had been completed

2.  37% (SD = 17%) of leg ulcer assessments had been completed
3.  63% (SD = 13%) of incontinence assessments had been completed.

However, it easy to see how these data can be used punitively rather then developmentally (Toms 1992).

It is understandable why documenting takes second place to giving care, especially when teams are short staffed. Toms (1992) felt that this outcome led to poor and inaccurate nursing records. However, district nursing document audits during the current author's fieldwork show that completion standards were more than acceptable, although some aspects of the records' content were unsatisfactory. It was assumed that the latter weakness was work pressure related rather than a lack of knowledge and skills. Nevertheless, this finding is important because not only workload implications but also of the medicolegal importance of accurate and complete clinical records. The Audit Commission (1999) concluded that, although poor documentation does not mean poor care, a worrying finding in their document audits was that some patients, receiving care from up to six different nurses, experience poor communication, fragmented care and duplication.

## Patient satisfaction

User-focused approaches, including patient satisfaction surveys, are popular, relatively simple and effective primary and community care quality measures. As with clinical audit, patient satisfaction surveys are commonly used by GPs. The Eli Lilly Consultation Satisfaction and Surgery Satisfaction Questionnaires are at the forefront because they are not only easy to use but also benchmarking is possible (Rink et al. 1996). Full instructions are included in the pack (Eli Lilly National Clinical Audit Centre 1992).

From satisfaction studies, Poulton and West (1994) and Kendall and Lissauer (2003) listed the issues most important to community patients and their carers:

*   Accessible and flexible appointments (one of the greatest dissatisfiers, particularly out of hours)
*   Minimal waiting
*   Carer information and education
*   Respite care
*   Privacy and confidentiality
*   Competent practitioners
*   Understanding professionals' roles
*   Continuity of care
*   Involvement.

Some of these featured heavily in the last Healthcare Commission PCT star-rating exercise (Stevenson et al. 2003), and in this chapter they are summarized from the PCT workforce planning and development (WP&D) database, where each PCT's data can be viewed (Table 5.2): www.health-careworkforce.org.uk

**Table 5.2** Patient satisfaction

| PCT/Band | Patient satisfaction | Complaints per 10 000 population |
|---|---|---|
| England | 3 | 1.7 |
| Three-star PCTs | 3 | 1.8 |
| ONS Band 1 PCTs | 3 | 3 |
| ONS Band 2 | 3 | 1.1 |
| ONS Band 3 | 3 | 1.8 |
| ONS Band 4 | 3 | 2.1 |
| ONS Band 5 | 3 | 1.5 |
| ONS Band 6 | 3 | 1.8 |
| Specimen Band 3 PCT | 3 | 6.2 |
| Specimen's percentile | NA | 98th |

The Healthcare Commission patient satisfaction score is a composite score ranging from 1 (poor) to 5 (good) The composite score is made up of patient satisfaction with: information and communication; cleanliness; comfort and friendliness; safe, quality and coordinated care. However, although the minimum and maximum scores were 1.2 and 4, respectively, the averages for the various bandings in Table 5.2 may not be sufficiently discriminatory. The number of complaints per 10 000 patients, on the other hand, has more precision.

Although patient satisfaction surveys are good for obtaining users' views, there are caveats. To get a representative view patients need to have been registered with a GP for at least 6 months and care should be taken to ensure that minority patients are included. Some patients have unrealistic expectations so they should be given opportunities to choose realistic options about changing services. Evaluators should compare professional and patients' perceptions of service quality and resist the view that patients are not experts and so have little to offer (Barriball and Mackenzie 1993; Poulton and West 1994; Audit Commission 1999; Proctor and Campbell 1999; Stevenson et al. 2003). Indeed, Rapport and Maggs (1997) noted the differences between patients and professionals' views of the same service:

- Patients felt well cared for
- Consultation times were long enough.

- But patients felt that they were the vulnerable partners and found it difficult to voice their needs (especially with GPs and Social Service staff).

Up to 98% of the patients in the UK are satisfied with their care but are less satisfied than their European counterparts. However, these data do not distinguish primary and secondary care (Rapport and Maggs 1997; Kendall and Lissauer 2003). Patient and carer satisfaction surveys in the literature include some unusual angles, e.g. studies on blurring health and Social Services showed that patients are worried about:

- where and how to obtain health services or Social Services
- what care will be received and the cost
- coordination, continuity and fragmentation.

Clearly, there is confusion about who is responsible when services are jointly provided. Triggle (2003) noted the agreements and disagreements between local authority and PCT managers about who is involved and what to ask patients. Concentrating on topics that can be measured, including visiting patterns, duration of contact, accessibility, information quality, education, continuity and location of care, and whether needs were met, may be the solution (Audit Commission 1999).

Focus groups, an alternative to patient-completed questionnaires, can be used to obtain what is important not only about the service but also for prioritizing the patients. In one study, 20 health-care and social care services were short-listed from 50 and, later, patients and practice staff were asked independently to say whether standards had been met for these prioritized services. Practice staff were given feedback about similarities and differences (the latter easily outnumbered similarities) between patients and professionals. Researchers noted resistance to service user surveys in some practices whereas others responded positively and acted on the findings (Stevenson et al. 2003).

# Community profiles

Population-based outcome measures, using caseload and community profiles, are preferred by some authors. This approach involves agreeing goals and aggregating data so that community health needs are understood and targets can be investigated. If measured annually they offer baselines that can be benchmarked to show improvements and sometimes the reasons for the improvement. Practitioners prefer these measures because group measures can overcome the distortion effects of small samples. Outcomes and related measures, appropriate for the community, can be selected and in some cases agreed with stakeholders. The main downside, on the other hand, is that population changes are long term and profiling may not be sensitive enough to detect improvements. Also, the community approach is time-consuming and potentially disparate if outcomes with nothing in common emerge (Kelsey 1995).

Whitmore et al.'s (1982a) study is dated but the outcomes and measures are still relevant:

- Proportion of school population screened (60% unscreened, 40% had problems about which GPs were unaware)
- Liaison meeting frequency and involvement (meetings rarely took place)
- Parent satisfaction (unhappiness that children's medication was being missed during school hours)
- Comparing parent's satisfaction with different professionals (satisfaction with GPs greater than satisfaction with school health service staff)
- Head teacher's first point of contact when there are health problems (school health service staff not the first port of call).

Contemporary data of this kind would be remarkably illuminating for workforce planning and development managers.

# Clinical audit

Clinical audit has been become an established method of measuring the quality of primary and community care. Anderson (1991) and Ong (1991) explain that primary and community audits fall into three categories:

1. Practice activity oriented such as prescribing rates, home visit dependability and punctuality
2. National standards-based work such as meeting diabetes mellitus protocol requirements
3. Staff behaviour-oriented such as practitioner–patient interaction when advice and technical care are provided coupled with professionals' understanding of the patients' needs.

General practitioners are active clinical auditors not least because of the Healthcare Commission star-rating requirements (Table 5.3).

Other audit topics include infection control, prescribing, and secondary and primary care interface issues (Proctor and Campbell 1999). The Audit Commission (1999) noted that clinical nursing audit was less successful because practitioners felt that it was 'done to them' and they rarely influenced the choice of audit topic. Also there are few evidence-based nursing standards against which to compare services, and the audit cycle was not completed, i.e. recommendations arising from the audit were rarely implemented or the service re-evaluated.

**Table 5.3** Practices with coronary heart disease audit data less than 1 year old

| PCT/Band | Percentage |
| --- | --- |
| England | 100 |
| Three-star PCTs | 100 |
| ONS Band 1 PCTs | 88 |
| ONS Band 2 | 100 |
| ONS Band 3 | 97 |
| ONS Band 4 | 98 |
| ONS Band 5 | 100 |
| ONS Band 6 | 100 |
| Specimen Band 3 PCT | 100 |
| Percentile | NA |

# Critical incidents

Critical incident reporting, such as drug-prescribing errors, can improve poor performance because staff learn from mistakes. However, complaints, for example, have been seen as policing rather than as improving services. It is important that problems are detected early and that managers do not resort to disciplinary measures, which cause autonomous practitioners to view critical incident-based measures suspiciously. Leach (1997), for example, noted how health visitors were pilloried when care was deemed suboptimal in cases of infant death. It is for these negative reasons that whistle blowing, an extension of critical incident reporting and a key component of clinical governance, may not be accepted by practitioners (Proctor and Campbell 1999; Hyde 2001).

# Workforce planning, development and quality from a professional group perspective

Another way of thinking about workforce planning and development, and efficiency and effectiveness, is to review data relating to specific staff groups. One obvious advantage is that workforce planning and development is staff group based and even multidisciplinary approaches can make use of staff group-specific data. However, modernization approaches such as *Liberating the Talents* (DoH 2002c) make professional group-oriented methods less useful because new work categories do not have enough benchmarks. In the short term at least, managers are going to rely on data from traditional working groups such as district nurses and community therapists.

The district nursing service cost £650m in 1999, 75–80% of which went on salaries. Differences in the number and mix of workers account for a 43% variation in PCT staff costs. One explanation is that recruitment and retention problems in certain parts of the UK mean that trust managers have to offer better grades to attract and keep practitioners. The influence of premature promotion on efficiency effectiveness is, however, unknown (Audit Commission 1999). One method is to relate staff numbers and mix to outcomes. However, Barriball and Mackenzie (1993) summarize the main community nursing outcome measurement problems as follows:

- Demonstration that a particular outcome was the result of an intervention (such as richer grade mix)
- Measurement of the outcomes of different categories of work such as prevention and continuing care
- Disentanglement of the contribution of staff groups such as community nurses in multidisciplinary team settings
- Demonstration that instruments have robust psychometric properties.

Probably as a result of these difficulties, the *Occupational Health Review* team (Anonymous 1994) was one of only a few research groups in the literature that explored the relationship between quality and staffing. Of their survey involving 393 nurses, 75% said that they had insufficient time to complete their work, blaming understaffing, cost cutting and a lack of managerial support. Worryingly, only 3% felt that the quality of community nursing care was satisfactory. Rink et al. (1996) also attempted to match quality and workload. Practitioners were asked to complete activity diaries and make a judgement each day about appropriate and inappropriate care (along 'Quality Pointer' lines). Diary findings were triangulated with a more objective measure, in this case a patient satisfaction survey. Klein and Tomlinson (1987b) showed that service quality suffered in localities that had high workloads. Piggott (1988) noted that health visitor interventions were sometimes 'make do' when workload peaked. She concluded that crisis-oriented working, clearly workload and staffing related, reduced service quality. However, Barkauskas' (1983) dated study showed that home visiting, which in itself is not always effective, contributed to excessive workloads. Clinics, it would seem, may be a better alternative although, as noted elsewhere, travel, access and patients who did not attend (DNAs) are important issues for those organizing and running clinic sessions.

Vetter et al. (1984) felt that practitioners may not be doing themselves favours. They suggested one area where staff can make differences to quality of life and life expectancy in elderly people, and yet health visitors, for example, spend disproportionately less time with this community patient group. Possibly as a result of incessant pressures on health visitors to show their worth, as professionals competing for resources, they are constantly being asked to provide evidence. Moreover, new pressures are emerging from *Liberating the Talents* (DoH 2002c) – an initiative that also offers many opportunities. Unfortunately, as Craig and Smith (1998) and Elkan et al. (2000b) point out, there is no simple evaluation framework that facilitates measuring a job such as health visiting which is relationship centred and with so many complex social processes. Also true of other community staff, health visitors keep a practical and experienced eye on families, and chronically ill and disabled people. Their pastoral role may not require specific interventions, so this almost invisible but important aspect of care is difficult to measure and certainly would not constitute an outcome. Pastoral care has to be articulated, however, possibly in the shape of proxy measures such as the number of visits to elderly people, for survival reasons (Latimer and Ashburner 1997).

According to the literature, it seems that evaluators have three choices:

1. disease, problem oriented
2. public health preventive
3. patient and community empowerment models.

Although Kelsey (1995) found 16 outcomes, three main measuring issues emerged:

1. The change must be related to health status.
2. Change must be measurable.
3. Change was directly attributable to work activity.

Despite the importance of relationship-centred health visiting, parents perceived health visitors as having a policing role – necessary and desirable but for other parents, not them! Preventive roles were scarcely appreciated or understood by parents. Encouragingly, on the other hand, parents said that health visitors were good at recognizing stress among family members. Worryingly, however, despite admitting the pressures of new motherhood, parents did not see their problems as relevant to any primary care professional – a situation that at least seems to have a public education message (Appleton 1994).

The influence of health visitor assistants on the quality of care has been explored in the literature. In one case, health visitors were surprised at the breadth and depth of nursery nurses' knowledge and skills, although there were gaps. Nevertheless, assistants released health visitors for higher-level work and consequently new services were being planned that included this new staff mix. On the downside, extra time and effort were needed to change the staff mix and establishments had to be increased so no savings were made. Also nursery nurses experienced a range of feelings from increased job satisfaction to anxiety, because they worked more closely with families (Seymour 1994).

Ebeid's (2000) localized primary and community nursing staff mix review led to a £10 000 saving by cutting senior posts and substituting roles. School nurses brought new skills whereas health-care assistants ran clinics without any productivity loss. Time was released, which allowed other team members to take on new work such as Sure Start. However, practitioners were worried that standards would fall if unpredictable work needing a senior practitioner, such as child protection, was not monitored. As in the case of health visitor assistants, the time and effort needed to bring about these staff-mix changes did not lead to savings.

Studies of practice nurse efficiency and effectiveness usually compare practice nurse and GP costs and quality, e.g. Heath (1994), Kendall and Lissauer (2003) noted that practice nurses performed as well as their GP colleagues although nurses saw fewer patients, which raised costs. Evidence showing that nurse practitioners and practice nurses are as efficient as their GP colleagues, on the other hand, is conflicting. Jenkins-Clarke et al. (1996) found no differences between the quality or the quantity of GP and practice nurse interventions. Importantly, patients did not mind whether they saw a nurse or a doctor as long as there was continuity of care and they were seen promptly. Hyde's more recent work (2001), a systematic review of trials comparing practice nurses/nurse practitioners with GPs, generates new and possibly more robust insights:

- Physical, emotional and social outcomes were no different.
- Patient satisfaction was high and the same for both professional groups. Children were more satisfied with practice nurses/nurse practitioners.
- Overall costs fell as far as comparisons could be made.
- Prescribing rates were lower.
- There was better access, stability and continuity for deprived area patients.
- Care was judged to be more holistic.
- Patients felt more informed.
- GP recruitment and retention problems were eased.
- Referrals and re-attending rates were no different.
- Consultations were longer but length could be reduced without compromising quality.

The extra time nurses spend, the social support they offer and the continuity of care they provide were welcomed by the patients (Kendall and Lissauer 2003). However, Martin (1987) felt that better outcomes depended on nurses' experience.

There are primary care developments in which staffing efficiency and effectiveness are especially important. Nurse and multidisciplinary team-led Personal Medical Service (PMS) pilots, for example, are delivering primary care services differently. They are community and patient focused, with in some cases patients as partners. Although these pilots may not suit all practice populations, those needing better access and more responsive services can benefit. PMSs are crucial for modernizing primary care services but they are proving costly. Worryingly, auditors found that some PMS staff had no financial data or controls despite these and other performance data being needed for evaluation (Tobin 2002; Walsh et al. 2003).

Seymour (1994) and Ebeid (2000) examined service quality specifically from a multidisciplinary and integrated working context. Dismantling professional barriers and multiskilling community teams appeared to:

- increase productivity
- reduce costs without reducing quality
- boost job satisfaction
- diminish inappropriate working
- accelerate service developments.

Managers, practitioners and lecturers, on the other hand, saw multiskilling as costly to set up or a threat to some professional groups, or were concerned about the education and training implications. Once again, evidence is conflicting. Researchers have shown that a richer staff mix does not automatically lead to better services because senior practitioners have a tendency to work inappropriately, spending less time in direct patient care. Conversely, dilute staff mix, which may follow unsystematic and irrational workforce planning and development, is likely to result in lower efficiency and effectiveness (Audit Commission 1992a).

## Conclusion

Primary and community care quality, addressed as efficiency (doing things right) and effectiveness (doing the right things) in the WP&D literature, offer valuable pointers generally and to WP&D specifically. The pressures on professionals to demonstrate their worth, as they compete for resources, has never been stronger. However, measuring effectiveness and efficiency in a WP&D context raises many challenges. The range of primary and community care quality measures in the literature is impressive but should a professional- or patient-centred stance be taken? Do structure, process and outcome criteria and measures have equal importance? Should Social Service outputs and outcomes be considered separately from NHS ones? To answer these questions managers consider efficiency and effectiveness in two main ways:

1. Professionally based evidence: the specific issues affecting practitioners.
2. Method based: the 'horses for courses' literature.

Few outcome data are collected centrally and there are even fewer bench-marks. This is frustrating because quality outcomes generate remarkable insights into workload and staffing. Recently, Healthcare Commission PCT star-rating data boosted the managers' armoury from which they can explore quality of care in a workload and staffing context. The Healthcare Commission data are not only growing but also breaking the mould. They include structure, process and outcome indicators, which means that researchers can begin to relate efficiency and effectiveness to the workforce. The latest outcome data are patient and employee satisfaction dominated because NHS user expectations are rising. Generally, patient satisfaction studies are a commonly used, simple (compared with the other methods at least) and effective way of measuring service quality. There are plenty of instruments and guidance in the literature (see Annotated bibliography, p. 167).

Clinical audit is another method that is Healthcare Commission moni-tored. However, audit has a mixed reception in the literature because it is less valuable to some primary and community care professionals and data are rarely explored in a workforce-planning context. Critical incidents are useful for evaluating primary and community care teams. However, they are viewed as a way of policing services rather than developing them. They rely on whis-tle blowing – something with which some professionals do not feel comfortable.

Comparing services against standards using patient records is another method that is well supported in the literature. This method is time-consuming and presents access problems to auditors because records are remotely located. Another problem is that most audits are process measures. Nevertheless, the armoury available to PCT managers is growing and little or no harm will befall those making forays into this vital component of work-force planning and development.

# CHAPTER SIX

# Education and training

## Introduction and background

Two main education and training issues emerge in the primary and community care workforce planning and development literature:

1. professional's responsibility for maintaining his or her knowledge and skills
2. manager's responsibility for service development by implementing modernization programmes.

Clearly, there is an expectation that managers and practitioners maintain and develop competency to practise by expanding knowledge and skills, recognizing personal accountability, engaging practitioners and clinical supervisors, and evaluating their performance. Clinical governance requirements expect community practitioners to base their practice on sound evidence including National Institute for Clinical Excellence (NICE) guidelines that emerge from systematic reviews, etc. (Department of Health or DoH 1993b; Hyde 2001).

However, as in most workforce planning and development (WP&D) issues there are challenges, e.g. even though information technology facilitates practice updating, Kendall and Lissauer (2003) estimate that practitioners wanting to keep abreast may need to read up to 19 articles each day. Clearly, this is unrealistic and, consequently, workforce development (separate from workforce planning) is important for several reasons including quality of care, personal development and job satisfaction (Hyde 2001).

## Curriculum

There are clear indications on important topics and how managers should be developing and supervising staff (DfES 2001; Lancaster and South Cumbria Education Training Consortium or and LSCETC 1998).

Fieldwork and literature reviewing by the author generated a substantial list of topics that community practitioners expect to see in the curriculum or developing into competencies (Atkin et al. 1994; Young 1997; Malone and Mackenzie 2000; Hyde 2001; DoH 2002c; Kendall and Lissauer 2003):

- Developing assistant nurses' knowledge and skills to care for elderly people and young chronic sick or mentally ill people in the community and those recovering from recent surgery.
- Developing registered practitioners' evidence-based knowledge and skills, ranging over assessment, investigation, diagnosis, treatment, care and rehabilitation, to deal with continuing care and chronic disease management (CDM) conditions such as asthma.
- Child health and protection.
- Nurse prescribing in GP-'thin' but practice nurse-'rich' primary care trusts (PCTs).
- Developing administrative staff's knowledge and skills for relieving community practitioners of clerical and related burdens in PCTs that are practice administrative staff 'rich'.
- Developing practice nurses' knowledge and skills to meet extended role implications of the new GMS contract and *Liberating the Talents* (DoH 2002c).
- Programmes to raise practitioners' personal safety awareness and methods for dealing with problems in areas with well above average crime rates in some PCTs, especially offences against the person.
- Education programmes for supervisors of isolated, autonomous practitioners.
- Cultural awareness programmes for community practitioners working in trusts with greater numbers of individuals from minority ethnic groups.
- Joint working with social services on elderly and child care, for example, which call for multidisciplinary courses.
- Managerial and administrative abilities such as management and leadership, achievement and motivation, communication, workload management, quality assurance and information management and technology (IM&T).
- Locating and using new knowledge.
- User involvement and shared decision-making.
- Social care issues including welfare rights and benefits.

It may be the nature of the literature reviewed but *Liberating the Talents'* three core functions – first contact, CDM and public health – were easily the most commonly mentioned. Most of the items listed above could be subsumed under these three headings.

# Competencies

Increasingly, the 14 topics above are being converted into competencies, aligned to National Service Frameworks (NSFs) such as the NSF for Diabetes and National Vocational Qualifications (NVQs), which form part of the skills escalator, pay and reward schemes (Cochrane et al. 2002; DoH 2002e; Kendall and Lissauer 2003). The value of competencies is underlined in the Future Healthcare Workforce literature, not least because they may reduce the burden of regulating practitioners. Competencies are defined as:

> The knowledge, skills and understanding to perform [at] work . . . .
>
> Cochrane et al. (2002, p. 34)

Trust managers and educators are particularly well placed to develop competencies for the community workforce (Cochrane et al. 2002). Indeed, Yole and Barrett (2003) set out a protocol to help managers develop appropriate competencies:

- Identify the gaps between services and staffing, especially specialist nurses and therapists.
- Develop the competencies for roles to fill the gaps and determine the contributions staff can make.
- Band the competencies:
  - effective care from assessment to evaluation
  - quality improvement and risk management
  - evaluation and research
  - inter- and intraprofessional team work
  - life-long learning
  - managing people, information, resources and the environment.

Each heading includes standards relating to knowledge, skills and attitudes, which Yole and Barrett tied to NVQs in the case of assistant grades. The outcomes were expected to clarify workers' expectations and responsibilities, match actual and expected roles, enhance career progression, and recognize and reward individual contributions.

Buckle and Gallen (2003) discuss the educational implications of first contact roles for practice nurses working under the supervision of GPs to an agreed list of competencies and protocols (e.g. triage and minor illness treatment). Protocols and guidelines are valuable support for isolated practitioners such as practice nurses because they are evidence based and show the practitioner his or her responsibilities and accountabilities (Latimer and Ashburner 1997). The practice nurse's first contact knowledge and skills are likely to be enhanced by external programmes organized by universities (Andrews 2004).

Wright (2002) listed those competencies for practice nurse assistants:

- Accountability
- Venepuncture
- Measuring vital signs
- Specimen collection and processing
- New patient registrations
- Participation in vaccination and immunization clinics
- Record keeping
- IM&T.

Staff in a number of agencies are working on primary and community care competencies. Once completed they can be accessed via the main Department of Health website.

## In-service education and training

In-service education also plays an important role in developing competencies. Jeffreys et al. (1995) noted that 51% of community staff in their survey were dissatisfied with their post-basic and in-service education and training, although the data were 10 years old. Practice nurses, for example, work not only in isolation but also in unprecedented change. These nurses deserve special attention because they have close ties with higher-level university education programmes, notably GP training schemes (DoH 2001b; Hyde 2001). Despite these issues, and possibly because practice nurse education and training are not mandatory, respondents in one survey said that education and training were at worst non-existent or at best inadequate. However, evidence in the literature can be conflicting, e.g. Hirst et al. (1998) noted that education innovation and developments could vary between practices. Only half of the practice nurse respondents in one census had attended a formal course. Nevertheless, their range of qualifications was impressive. Only a minority held extended roles certificates such as care of patients with diabetes and asthma (Atkin et al. 1994; Hyde 2001). In 1994, 61% of practice nurses in the Atkin study experienced problems because study leave was refused as a result of lack of staff in the small general practices in which they worked. Ten per cent had not had one study day in the preceding year but the average paid and unpaid study days were six per year.

Community nurses also reported varying levels of education and training although findings from surveys today are likely to be different because of clinical governance and PCT interventions (LSCETC 1998; Hyde 2001). Indeed PCT managers in recent interviews with the author had growing faith in local education and training programmes. They felt, for example, that NVQs were a boon to health-care assistant development, especially because services were likely to become dependent on these staff. On the whole, despite work pressures and tight budgets, managers felt that they maintained good standards of staff development and met compulsory staff education obligations. However, they were conscious of up-and-coming changes such as diminishing part-time courses and their reliance on staff goodwill for attending sessions during lunch breaks. Indeed, recent evidence shows that staff personal development time is suffering (McDonald et al. 1997). Jenkins-Clarke and Carr-Hill's (2001) survey, for example, showed that 65% of community practitioners, especially health visitors, worked unpaid overtime – 15% higher than hospital nurses' unpaid contribution. PCT managers in the author's fieldwork were determined not to let professional development time slip because of its positive influence on job satisfaction, recruitment and retention. Clearly, there's a trade-off between clinical and educational commitments.

The Department of Health, noting many of the variations summarized above, is determined to streamline education structure and process to ensure that demarcations between professional groups are broken down (DoH 2001a). One of *Liberating the Talents'* aims is to give practitioners greater freedom while still part of multidisciplinary teams. To achieve practitioner autonomy the Department of Health (2002c) explains the following:

- Managers need to 'let go' of their staff. Frontline workers, for example, should manage budgets and staffing.
- The frontline workforce needs to be empowered.
- A no-blame culture needs to be encouraged.
- Champions with drive and enthusiasm should become service leaders.
- Service priorities need clarification.
- Staff development time needs protection.
- Best practice and innovation require accessible evidence databases.
- Multiprofessional networks need to be created.

There is a risk that assistant grades may, however, get a raw deal despite the increasingly important role that they will play (Kendall and Lissauer 2003, p. xvi):

> The needs of the non-professional qualified workforce have not been given sufficient priority . . . the lack of training support for this group of staff is a particular cause for concern. It's recommended that the NHS universities should make courses a priority. Also the lack of a common language or competencies for vocational professional occupations makes the transition from support worker to professional more difficult than it need be.

One reason for the problem, as Chalmers and Kristajanson (1989) noted, is the tension between education and practice. They felt that educators and practitioners were not 'singing from the same hymn sheet'. They also believed that the balance of health promotion, prevention and treatment is not right and that there needed to be curriculum and practice changes. One way innovation might be brought about is through the following (DoH 2002b, 2002c):

- Analysing the community's needs
- Mapping the services that are currently provided
- Bringing stakeholders together, including primary and secondary carers
- Identifying the service gaps
- Assessing practitioners' knowledge and skills
- Setting clear aims and objectives and means to measure them
- Checking that the plan accords with the trust's and Workforce Development Confederation's priorities and secure sponsorship
- Developing practitioners' clinical roles.

Clearly, these items have to be considered in a modernized, competency-based service, which also recognizes the mentoring and supervision strengths and weaknesses.

## Supervision, mentorship and appraisal

The complex nature of primary and community health care demands that all practitioners should be supported through clinical supervision. This enables staff to keep their practice under review, and develop and be accountable for their work (DoH 1993b). Mentoring and supervision, which are sensitive to team size and mix, are important education and training issues for the following reasons (Audit Commission 1992a; Lochead 1994; Buckingham and Wilson 1997; Latimer and Ashburner 1997; Nicholson 1998; Hyde 2001; Walsh et al. 2003):

- They were made mandatory through clinical governance.
- Extended and new roles have been created.
- Managers can be responsible for up to 60 community staff, dispersed throughout the community. There is a risk that these staff work not only out of sight but also without supervision – unaccountable and unsupported.
- Reflection with a supervisor can enhance personal development and quality of care.

District nurses in one comprehensive study were asked to rate the value of clinical supervision (Hurst et al. 2002) (Table 6.1). Interestingly, unsupervised nurses' ranking was similar but their levels of agreement were lower.

**Table 6.1** Value of clinical supervision

| Element | Agreement (%) |
| --- | --- |
| Helps practice reflection | 92 |
| Improves confidence | 84 |
| Facilitates practice development | 84 |
| Relieves stress | 74 |
| Identifies development needs | 69 |
| Promotes professional standards | 65 |
| Raises job satisfaction | 60 |
| Focuses on innovation | 51 |
| Increases understanding of roles | 45 |
| Encourages interdisciplinary working | 38 |

However, there are problems. Not all GPs and senior nurses are keen to supervise because it takes them away from their clinical duties. Also, it takes time to develop trust between mentors and practitioners from different professional backgrounds (Hyde 2001). One study of allied health professional (AHP) supervisor:student ratios (LSCETC 1998) showed wide variations: anywhere from 1:1 to 1:5.7 professionals to students; clearly the latter ratio would be difficult to operate in the community. The Audit Commission (1999) noted a variable and worsening situation. The number of fieldwork teachers in the community in their studies had fallen by 8% in the 3 years to 2000. It is not clear, however, whether, this fall is recruitment and retention related or caused by a lack of managerial commitment. Clinical governance, notably continuing professional development, mentoring and clinical supervision, requires a richer staff mix for satisfactory supervisor and supervisee ratios. In addition, basic nurse education seems to be constantly under review and the time student nurses spend in community care settings is likely to change. Managers value student placements but the degree to which students demand time from staff or, conversely, contribute to the workload can vary. These issues should cause managers to review clinical supervision regularly.

Similarly, the number of health-care assistants and their roles are expanding. As noted earlier, these workers make a valuable contribution to community care (Lochead 1994; McIntosh et al. 2000; Richards et al. 2000). However, diluting the workforce raises supervision problems. More staff have to be supervised and there are fewer supervisors – especially important when the workforce is geographically widespread (McIntosh et al. 2000). Indeed, almost a third of community practitioners in one study felt that their supervisory duties were increasing (Wright 1998). If the qualified to assistant grade ratios continue to be diluted, it is probable that highly skilled operatives will become merely delegators and supervisors (Heath 1994).

Despite investment in expensive education programmes some practitioners were not confident in their abilities (e.g. prescribing). Consequently, important new services could not be established. However, robust supervision and mentorship allowed new services to work, which resulted in significant efficiency and effectiveness improvements. This not only results in a good return on the PCT's investment but also makes better use of service managers' and leaders' expertise as practitioners to lead service changes (Hyatt 2003).

Appraisal is closely aligned to supervision and mentorship and, although adding to the senior practitioner's 'administrative' burden, appraisal can benefit the service. Appraisal ensures that personal development plans are up to date, which identify the development and educational needs that are related to primary and community care. Appraisal also keeps isolated practitioners more involved (Latimer and Ashburner 1997; Hyde 2001).

## Conclusion

Workforce planning and workforce development are sometimes used synonymously in the literature. However, similar to skill mix and grade mix they are different, equally important and a powerful combination. Workforce development is primarily about boosting practitioners' knowledge and skills so that staffing configurations are given a chance to work. Separating workforce development from workforce planning helps PCT managers distinguish staff from skills shortage. Workforce development is strongly tied to workforce planning, especially when staff mix is changed and practitioners' roles are extended or altered in other ways as a result of new services or policies. Workforce development falls into three categories:

1. what staff development topics need to be covered
2. how topics are taught and learned
3. supervision, mentoring and appraisal.

It has never been more important for practitioners to keep abreast of health-care and social care policy and practice developments. Indeed, recently clinical governance made continuing professional development and supervision mandatory. Specifically, PCT workforce, socioeconomic and morbidity data, examined in the context of national policies, raise several workforce development issues. These blend well with a rich source of topics and guidance in the literature, which add additional insight (see Annotated bibliography, page 167). The range is wide but CDM as a workforce development topic, as the Evercare sites show, is popular.

Older surveys show that up to 80% of primary and community staff were dissatisfied with their education and training, which means that PCT managers probably inherited under-funded and under-committed staff development programmes. Some critics point out that primary and community care services and education are only slowly being aligned. However, higher education centres are steadily creating programmes that prepare practitioners for their rapidly changing roles, while developing Workforce Development Confederation and universities continuing professional development programmes is important.

Supervision and mentorship are increasingly significant in primary and community care, not least because of clinical governance and expanding practitioner roles. Linked to appraisal they assist personal development. However, staff mix in some PCTs makes adequate supervision and mentorship a challenge, e.g. the specimen PCT examined regularly throughout the book has 50% fewer district nurses than its ONS Band 6 or three-star PCT counterparts. Clearly, supervision is another important and challenging workforce development area and is taken up again Chapter 7.

# CHAPTER SEVEN

# Recruitment and retention

## Introduction and background

Today's NHS staff shortages can be traced back to the 1990s when internal market policies encouraged managers to regulate workforce size and mix in an over-cautious way. Consequently, the numbers in training halved and as a result of the 'slowing oil tanker' effect, the full effects are now being felt. Although employee numbers increased in recent years, there were still 6000 fewer trainees in the year 2000 than there were in 1990 (Buchan and Edwards 2000). As a measure of the seriousness of workforce supply, 85% of trusts in one survey experienced recruitment and retention problems (Collins et al. 2000).

However, after concerted efforts the numbers returning to or joining the NHS have increased by 1.9% since 1999 and are expected to climb 25% by 2009. Similarly, the number (head counts not whole-time equivalents or WTEs) of consultants rose by 4.7%, scientific and technical staff by 3.4%, allied health professionals (AHPs) by 3% and GPs by 1.3%. Nurses' education places have increased by 30% since 1992 and the number of applicants by 35%. However, at 17% attrition is unacceptably high. Apart from GPs these data relate to the NHS broadly, and it is not clear how many of these are leaving or joining primary and community care (Davies 2000a; Department of Health or DoH 2001a).

The government has set stringent staffing and personnel targets, but providing data and algorithms to help primary care trust (PCT) workforce planners determine the most appropriate workforce size and mix can easily be fruitless if the employee supply side dries up. Achieving the right workforce size and mix means balancing supply-side and demand-side forces and, consequently, the supply side cannot be ignored (DoH 2002b) Unsurprisingly, clear recruitment and retention problem themes emerge from the literature and both recruitment and retention are addressed directly and indirectly in this section.

# The greying and shrinking NHS workforce

The NHS workforce is 'greying' and workforce planning is increasingly age sensitive. One in seven or 150 000 NHS workers is 50 years or older and the number of older, experienced professionals approaching retirement age, coupled with those who intend to retire early (up to 100% in some professional groups), compounds the problem.

Up to 5000 nurses leave the NHS each year, and this number is expected to double in the next decade because nurses are eligible to retire 5 years earlier than most female workers. Consequently, up to 1 in 10 nurses is contemplating retirement (Seccombe and Smith 1997; Buchan 1998, 1999; Audit Commission 1999; Mathie and McKinley 1999; Snell 2000a; Jenkins-Clarke and Carr-Hill 2001; Bosma and Higgins 2002; Davies 2000a; Fatchett and Gleeson 2002; Mathie 2002; Cole 2003a; Sibbald et al. 2003).

- The mean age of all nurses is 39 years whereas the district nurses' mean is 45 years. One-quarter of district nurses and one-third of health visitors (*n* = 50 000) are aged 50 years or older, an increase from 19% to 26% in recent years.
- Some 12% of practice nurses are aged 55 years or older.
- Community-nursing assistants are the oldest primary and community care staff group. However, health-care assistants (of which there are proportionally more) are younger.
- A third of GPs are aged over 50 years. Asian practitioners are disproportionately represented in this group, many of whom work in deprived areas. In one regional study, half of the GP workforce planned to retire by 2005. They blamed workload and job dissatisfaction for their desire to leave.
- Up to 25 000 NHS staff retire early each year on health grounds at a cost of £1bn, a figure, although falling, deemed excessive and costly. For some professional groups, however, the numbers are rising disproportionately.
- GPs are one staff group that is short of workers. Consequently, a target of 2000 more GPs has been set for 2004. However, unfilled practitioner vacancies doubled recently, which is compounded by the falling number of applicants. At 53.2 GPs per 100 000 population, one region with a 10% vacancy factor in the present study was 400 practitioners short.
- The pool of non-working nurses, from which trust managers draw, is shrinking and by 2030 the workforce will be 10% smaller than it is currently.
- Nationally, there is a 1% shortfall in health-care trainee recruitment and university admission department staff report, for some courses, that they have not built a cohort in several years. As a result, education cohorts increasingly feature older students.

In short, the number of nurses under 30 has halved in recent years and by 2005 there will be 30% fewer women between 16 and 24 years than two decades ago. These data are depressing but worse is that the loss of the most experienced practitioners is increasing. Primary and community managers are facing one of their biggest challenges and these supply-side problems could easily stifle any demand-side solutions.

# Vacancies

Vacancy data provide useful recruitment and retention insights, e.g. Davies (2000a) and Meadows et al. (2000) noted that the 3-month NHS vacancy rate ranged between 2% and 3.9% although the Department of Health vacancy survey showed hotspots with up to 16% vacancies. The national vacancy rate for nursing was 2.9% (SD = 1.2) whereas the district nursing percentage was lower at 1.3% and health visitors 1.8%. The latter data offer some comfort. The data for 2002 are summarized in Table 7.1, which shows interesting but logical variations between PCTs in different Office for National Statistics (ONS) bands.

**Table 7.1** Primary care trust (PCT) personnel variables

| PCT/Band | Unemployment (%) | Nurse vacancies (%) | AHP vacancies (%) | Full:part-time ratio | Staff satisfaction | Sickness absence (%) | Improving working lives |
|---|---|---|---|---|---|---|---|
| England | 3 | 1.6 | 4.2 | 1:1.39 | 3[a] | 4.1 | 2 |
| Three-star PCTs | 3 | 1.4 | 3.9 | 1.42 | 3 | 4 | 2 |
| ONS Band 1 PCTs | 5.7 | 6.4 | 6.7 | 1.33 | 2.8 | 4.5 | 2 |
| ONS Band 2 | 4.1 | 1.3 | 4.1 | 1.34 | 3 | 4.3 | 2 |
| ONS Band 3 | 3.8 | 1.3 | 5.1 | 1.34 | 3 | 4.1 | 2 |
| ONS Band 4 | 3.1 | 2 | 5.9 | 1.37 | 3 | 4.2 | 2 |
| ONS Band 5 | 2.3 | 2.2 | 4.7 | 1.46 | 3 | 3.7 | 2 |
| ONS Band 6 | 3 | 1.3 | 3.8 | 1.39 | 3 | 4.2 | 2 |
| Specimen Band 3 PCT | 5.3 | 1.6 | 3.9 | 1.42 | 3 | 2.3 | 2 |
| Specimen's percentile | 93rd | 50th | 35th | 70th | NA | 7th | |

[a] 5 = best rating; 2 = standard has been met.
AHP, allied health professional.

The shortage of certain staff groups and the diminishing pool from which employers are recruiting, notably the implications of a 7% medical practitioner and 10% nursing shortage, are severely affecting the supply of health-care professionals (Jenkins-Clarke 1997; Jenkins-Clarke and Carr-Hill 2001). Rural areas seemed to be suffering the most. In one study, despite extra funding, 7% of general practices had vacancies and 13% of their unfilled GP posts had been vacant for at least 3 months. Even before this worsening trend, some rural practices fell well short of the national GP recruitment target (Moody 2003). Nursing vacancies and the bank/agency/overtime replacement data are equally worrying, but they relate to the NHS and cannot easily be separated into primary, community and secondary care (Davies 2000a).

Recent Department of Health vacancy data show that AHP recruitment and retention is suffering to the extent that warning bells are ringing. Indeed, this professional group shows the greatest variation in Table 7.1. Managers in the author's PCT study raised important AHP supply-side issues, e.g. therapy managers increasingly were competing with the private sector, which had several negative effects on the NHS workforce. Some AHPs preferred to work for private agencies as a result of the variety of work settings and the flexibility that agencies offered. On the down side, agency staff are not only costly but also inadvertently diminish continuity of care, which staff in substantive posts provide. The less popular care groups, such as elderly people, were becoming even less attractive to NHS and agency AHP staff. One consequence of these problems is that PCT physiotherapy services in the author's study were under-established, which meant that more work was falling on to care assistants' shoulders.

Meadows et al. (2000) examined the public's view of nursing. Despite consistently negative media reporting, nursing is viewed positively by the public. The job is seen as broad ranging and expanding its role, and as having a growing autonomy. However, younger people are less convinced about nursing as a career. As discussed elsewhere, potential employees are worried about workplace violence, and nurses' status, hard work and low pay.

The precariousness of vacancy and related data in the case study PCT in Table 7.1 varies, despite some attractive features, such as:

- good and relatively inexpensive housing
- the availability of broad clinical experiences
- perceptions that the trust is a good place to work; PCT managers confirmed that there were more vacant posts than applicants as a result of:
  - two large teaching hospitals within easy travelling distance, which usually had first refusal
  - the pool from which senior practitioners were drawn was shrinking locally and even therapy service managers were being head hunted
  - career progression was limited in the smaller services and is reducing nationally as health services become less hierarchical
  - the clinical grading policy in the 1990s had damaged staff satisfaction (Buchan and Edwards 2000), although negative influences were diminishing

- although most primary and community practitioners are committed, full of energy, and willing to take on new roles and extend their practice, others are jealous, suspicious or lack trust in their colleagues and resist change (Bosma and Higgins 2002).

Unemployment data in Table 7.1 are only a crude indicator of worker participation. Even then data may be relevant only to certain staff groups such as local nursing assistant recruitment.

## Turnover

Hyatt (2003) felt that competition between PCTs is increasing and that financial reward may not be enough to recruit and retain staff:

> More nursing and more support staff are needed to deliver a safe and effective service. It is unlikely that the ability to recruit more staff would also help to stem the tide of staff who leave because of insupportable pressures.
>
> Meadows et al. (2000, p. 60)

Management styles may need to change so that leadership can develop and teams be democratically run. The implications were well articulated by managers interviewed by the author. Typically, managers confirmed pressures that influenced not only workload but also morale, recruitment and retention, which have been summarized in this chapter. Data from one PCT in the author's study showed a staff turnover rate at 21%, 7% having left for personal reasons. The ratio of starters to leavers across the PCTs studied by the author was as shown in Table 7.2.

**Table 7.2** Ratio of starters to leavers across the primary care trusts

| Professional group | Leaver:starter ratio |
| --- | --- |
| Nurses | 1:8 |
| HCAs | 1:5 |
| AHPs | 1:2 |

AHPs, allied health professionals; HCAs, health-care assistants.

These ratios vary among PCTs but they are higher than the private sector. The turnover rate in Davies' (2000a) study, for example, equated to 6.3%, whereas Noakes and Johnson's (1999) recorded staff turnover at 14.3%. Clearly, some areas experience turnover rates greater than the public sector (13.9%). The author's data from 323 general practices showed the turnover rates (Table 7.3).

**Table 7.3** Turnover rates in general practices

| Staff | Percentage turnover |
|-------|---------------------|
| General practitioner | 4.2 |
| Practice nurse | 12 |
| Manager | 8 |
| Administrative staff | 13 |

Elsewhere, Sibbald et al.'s (2003) trend analysis showed that 8% more GPs said they would quit in 2002 compared with the percentage 5 years earlier. Reasons included: (1) a naturally ageing workforce and (2) ethnic minority status and job dissatisfaction. Reasons for staying, on the other hand, included job satisfaction and the cost of raising children (implying that a substantial income was needed). Staggeringly, general practice managers, on average, will need to recruit 11 staff in each practice during the next 5 years just to stand still.

The practice nursing workforce also cannot afford to suffer losses because of the following (Noakes and Johnson 1999):

- 'greying' practice nurse workforce
- uncompetitive rates of pay
- inferior professional development programmes and the skills deficit
- higher turnover
- doubts that the *Agenda for Change* will be honoured
- managers needing to draw on the wider community workforce to fill the gaps.

# Job satisfaction

Healthcare Commission star rating data include staff job satisfaction indicators so PCT managers can benchmark themselves against three-star (and ONS similar) trusts. These data have been summarized in Table 7.1 and can be downloaded from www.healthcareworkforce.org.uk.

If health-care professionals, notably AHPs, have the upper hand (the sellers' market syndrome) and the workforce is shrinking then job satisfaction is something that PCT managers increasingly judge to be important for recruiting and retaining staff (Buchan and Edwards 2000). Traynor and Wade's (1992a, 1992b) data, although 10 years old, offer useful pointers. They surveyed 1500 primary and secondary care staff and asked them about five job satisfaction issues. The job aspects causing most dissatisfaction (in rank order) were:

1. Workload: 38%
2. Education and training: 37%
3. Pay and prospects: 32%
4. Professional support: 17%
5. Overall job satisfaction: 21%
6. Personal job satisfaction: 13%.

Later, Goodman (1996) found that 54% of the community workforce were dissatisfied with their jobs and 80% gave work pressure as the reason. This top ranking issue may be becoming more of a problem because the *Occupational Health Review* (Anonymous 1994) researchers noted that rising workload, particularly administrative, easily diminished any satisfaction gained from direct patient care – one of the most enjoyable parts of a practitioner's daily work. The negative issues causing community practitioners to leave for better-paid jobs that gave more satisfaction (Meadows et al. 2000) included the profession's:

- perceptions of current primary and community care developments, which are further threatening their jobs
- view that they are unseen and undervalued
- feeling that they are under-used
- dissonance over the way that their traditional work (highly valued) is being taken over by a plethora of new responsibilities, particularly managerial and administrative.

Other job satisfaction surveys unearthed some equally worrying findings (Whitmore et al. 1982a; Anonymous 1994; Seccombe and Smith 1997; Buchan 1999; Buchan and Edwards 2000; Collins et al. 2000; Meadows et al. 2000; Shields and Ward 2001; Hyatt 2003):

- Surveys showed that anywhere from 27% to 86% of staff were seriously thinking of leaving because of low pay, lack of resources, covering unfilled vacancies, work stress or poor recognition.
- Practitioners were unhappy with managers who failed to take action and resolve safety, discrimination and racism problems.
- Only one-third was satisfied with pay and only half liked their working hours.
- Fewer than 21% were happy with career progression, compounded when practitioners were unable to use newly acquired skills from specialist courses because of workload and the flatter, less hierarchical structure in which they worked.
- Many were dissatisfied with accommodation, crèche and leisure facilities.
- A worryingly low number (30%) were happy with their workload and staff levels.

- Most were unhappy that grade mix had been diluted in the search for efficiency.
- Males, ethnic-minority group members, and less qualified and mental health practitioners were the least satisfied.
- Older nurses felt burned out and were less likely to re-train for different roles that are part of flexible retirement schemes.
- Older, married staff with families, and those in innovative jobs, paediatric, community and primary care staff, were more satisfied.

PCT managers can take some comfort from the last point. Managers interviewed by the author agreed with most reasons in the literature and were taking action. They felt that staff job satisfaction among their subordinates was high but some felt they were beginning to lose the workforce's goodwill. On the upside, managers felt that the trusts' pay structure, workplace accommodation, job variation, staff development and IM&T developments had improved job satisfaction. Buchan (1998) offers other clues, i.e. mature nurses move to primary and community services because of the autonomy that this sector offers. However, because they are older and have different attitudes, they may need different incentives to stay in the job (Buchan 1999).

Workplace violence has always been a problem for health-care professionals and, although no evidence relating violence to recruitment and retention was located in the literature, job safety is likely to affect sick leave and retention. Unsurprisingly, therefore, writers are turning their attention to problems and solutions.

Data in Table 7.4 show that up to 14% of people are victims of crime – events to which primary and community care workers are susceptible, including assaults, theft, burglaries and car crimes. The variation in incidents is staggering and the case study trust has one of the worst crime rates of all the PCTs.

**Table 7.4** Crime vulnerability

| PCT/Band | Crimes per 1000 people |
|---|---|
| England | 44 |
| Three-star PCTs | 40 |
| ONS Band 1 PCTs | 102 |
| ONS Band 2 | 55 |
| ONS Band 3 | 72 |
| ONS Band 4 | 39 |
| ONS Band 5 | 33 |
| ONS Band 6 | 37 |
| Specimen Band 3 PCT | 130 |
| Specimen's percentile | 98th |

Specifically, there were 95 500 NHS workplace violence incidents in 2002. Nurses are five times more likely to be attacked at work and community practitioners working in inner city areas are particularly at risk from drug-related crime (Meadows et al. 2000; Cole 2003b). Between a third and a half of the nurses surveyed said that they had been assaulted in the preceding 12 months and the average incidence among community staff was two assaults per year. However, 4% suffered weekly attacks (Anonymous 1994; Cole 2003b). Patients and carers were predominantly responsible for these attacks, which were more likely to go unreported. Community staff are more vulnerable because help is slower to arrive and staff are working in strange territory. Violence is predicted to increase as community work expands, particularly as the out-of-hours programmes in the new General Medical Service (GMS) contract change (Cole 2003b).

Apart from education and training, only a third of nurses in the *Occupational Health Review* (Anonymous 1994) study received guidance for dealing with workplace violence. Cole (2003b) lists ways for dealing with the problem:

- Defining 'assault' and developing active, easier reporting and prosecuting procedures
- Listing known troublemakers
- Rapid police response procedures
- Recording photographs, next-of-kin, car details and known movements of lone and vulnerable workers
- Better street lighting and CCTV in problem areas
- Pairing and escorting schemes
- Strengthened car locks
- Risk assessments.

Trust managers may not have a workplace violence infrastructure in place (Cole 2003b), for example, and worryingly only half of the nurses in the *Occupational Health Review* survey (Anonymous 1994) said that their employers had schemes in which staff were paired in high-risk areas.

## Education and training issues

Although Chapter 6 explored the issue in detail, post-basic education and training regularly crop up as a job satisfaction issue and, therefore, are worth rehearsing. Indeed, there were several articles, books and reports that discussed education and training in a recruitment and retention context, and the issues were wide ranging, e.g. Meadows et al. (2000) underlined the importance of access to high-quality, flexible programmes. They also decried the lack of personal development time in the NHS.

The number of practitioners with district nursing qualifications is falling (Audit Commission 1999), whereas the author's interviews with PCT managers showed the effects these demographic and professional issues were having, notably a shortage of specialists in the field, including:

- nurse leaders
- infection control and tuberculosis specialists
- tissue viability practitioners
- continence advisers
- public health experts
- stroke rehabilitation staff
- multiple sclerosis rehabilitation specialists
- elderly care staff.

Hirst et al. (1998) looked at training general practices and noted that they were more likely to recruit and retain practitioners. Yole and Barrett (2003) found that competencies, which clarified the roles of community practitioners and their assistants, also improved recruitment and retention.

## Succession planning and other solutions

As a result of demographic and related problems facing NHS managers, succession planning, for which the NHS is heavily criticized (Buchan 1999), is becoming harder to achieve. Consequently, several recently produced documents offer guidance for improving PCT recruitment and retention (Noakes and Johnson 1999; DoH 2000b; Meadows et al. 2000; NHS Executive 2000b; National Primary and Care Trust Organisation or NatPaCT 2002a):

- Coordinated personnel policies
- Staff turnover, time-out recording and reporting
- Exit interviews with all leavers
- International recruitment strategies
- Return to practice programmes
- Family friendly policies:
  - flexible working
  - childcare facilities
  - flexible retirement
- Workplace equality and diversity:
  - equal opportunities policy and monitoring
  - tackling student hardships
- High-quality personnel advice and expertise:
  - good access
  - written standards

- Employment practices that support retention:
  - monitoring practice
  - external accreditation such as Investors in People
- Supervision, appraisal and personal development plans for all staff:
  - policies that cover staff in both substantive and temporary posts
  - staff involvement, partnerships and fora in which experiences can be discussed
- Occupational health
  - written service level agreements between occupational health service and PCT for all employees
  - formal provision of consultant occupational health physician advice
  - multidisciplinary occupational health strategic planning
- Securing the right size of workforce with the right skills to deliver fast, convenient and accessible primary and community care:
  - Integrated Health Improvement Plans, service workforce and financial frameworks (SWaFF)
  - scoping the existing workforce
  - forward planning
  - options for developing the future workforce
  - an overall workforce action plan
  - encouraging professionals to honour a statutory body's code of practice and supporting practitioners whose practice is below standard while inculcating a no-blame culture
- Encouraging practitioners to stay without penalizing them financially. If a post-retirement job is lower paid then pension entitlement is preserved.

The checklist is a tall order for any PCT manager. Nevertheless, monitoring bodies expect to see relevant strategies in trusts' annual workforce plans. Other, recently issued guidance for improving job satisfaction, recruitment and retention and succession planning sets out solutions to help managers use the checklist (Buchan 1998; DoH 1999b, 2000b, 2001a, 2002b; NHS Executive 2000a, 2000b; Meadows et al. 2000; Leeds Community and Mental Health Services Teaching NHS Trust or LCMHT 2001; Bosma and Higgins 2002; Cole 2003a; Moody 2003; Sibbald et al. 2003):

- Workforce age profiling.
- Non-age discrimination policies and flexible retirement schemes such as job wind-down that includes less demanding work for those approaching retirement.
- Registers of retired staff willing to work temporarily (e.g. during holidays).
- Age-oriented career planning and career break policies.
- Incentive schemes that encourage workers to stay beyond 60 years.

- Enhanced continuous professional development programmes.
- National Vocational Qualifications for health-care assistants.
- Cadet schemes for school leavers.
- University and Workforce Development Confederation collaborating to create flexible health-care professional education programmes that enable, for example, in-house education and training.
- Multidisciplinary teams and other, new ways of doing things.
- Career start schemes for GPs with special interests.
- Overseas recruitment.

Davies' (2000a) study showed that (in order of popularity) the reasons why nurses return to work are:

- part-time and flexible working
- refresher courses
- help with childcare
- better pay.

Return to practice is singled out in the literature as a key recruitment and retention variable. These need to be free of charge, and include supervision, mentorship and crèche facilities followed by flexible working on return to work. These are important if the 9000 nurses who have returned to the NHS in 2000 are to remain. Enticing senior staff to remain is mainly monetary: seniority payments; cost of living supplements; providing housing in London and the south east; and childcare provision (DoH 2001a). Housing stock is proving to be a challenge because NHS accommodation was reduced by 55% in the 1990s, affecting those trust managers with the severest staff shortages (NHS Executive 2000b). Despite this realization there is still an 'efficiency savings culture' in the NHS that is eroding budgets. Trust managers are being judged on their ability to trim costs (Meadows et al. 2000).

Where service gaps remain the Department of Health (2001a) is developing NHS Professionals – an in-house agency with a database and mechanisms to call in nurses at short notice. This new service is designed to reduce agency bills. The initiative of the NHS Professionals attempts to match demand and supply when trust managers struggle to recruit or there has been a sickness–absence surge, which forces managers to use agencies for replacing staff – running at £300m annually. The new flexi-pool scheme has several benefits. Apart from NHS equivalent rates of pay and compensation if work is cancelled at short notice, staff have the usual employee benefits such as joining the NHS pension scheme. There is paid annual leave and an occupational health scheme. Finally, staff have the opportunity to participate in continuing professional development programmes (NHS Executive 2000b). Obeid (1997) pre-empted NHS Professionals with a scheme designed for primary and community care. In her locality the demand for district nursing was growing and, apart from practice nursing, recruitment and retention was a problem. Her solution was a peripatetic practitioner who combined primary and community nursing. Importantly, there were common education and training programmes. Similarly, Cochrane et al. (2002) and Kendall and Lissauer (2003) recommended a new community health-care practitioner – a generic worker who would not need protracted education and training, and a role that also widens the entry gate, which might attract more workers into the NHS. The downside is the different conditions of employment experienced by practice and mainstream community nurses, when GPs might be reluctant to let practice nurses expand their roles (Obeid 1997). *Liberating the Talents* (DoH 2002c) is likely to crystallize these issues.

## *Improving Working Lives*

Current NHS personnel policy and practice has four pillars (Meadows et al. 2000; NHS Workforce Taskforce et al. 2002):

1. Making the NHS a three-star employer
2. Skills escalator for career progression
3. Improving staff morale
4. Building personnel management knowledge and skills.

Specifically, the *Improving Working Lives* report (Meadows et al. 2000; NHS Executive 2000a; DoH 2001a) was written to help personnel and other managers modernize their services and maintain the four pillars. In the report authors noted that staff perform best when work and home life are balanced. Feeling valued and receiving both clinical and educational support from employers, improving the employee's autonomy and control, and clear working protocols are also important (Meadows et al. 2000; Collins et al. 2000). Autocratic managers, on the other hand, who fail to deal with staff shortages and relieve work overload, were reasons why staff left. As raised earlier, role conflict, poor remuneration, lack of resources and isolated working were also important elements that cause job dissatisfaction, especially in the community workforce. It is clear from the Department of Health and other guidance that trusts are expected to appoint a manager specifically responsible for *Improving Working Lives*, with clear aims and objectives for:

- flexi-time working
- annual hours
- reduced hours options
- crèche support for children when parents are working; similarly carer support schemes

- career breaks
- flexible retirement.

Progress and problems meeting these objectives have to be monitored and reported to strategic health authorities (NHS Executive 2000b; DoH 2001a; NHS Workforce Taskforce et al. 2002). In 2004, PCTs were rated on their performance, which contributed to overall star ratings (see the PCT workforce planning and development [WP&D] database on www.healthcareworkforce.org.uk).

Sibbald et al.'s (2003) study provides other clues for *Improving Working Lives*. As raised earlier, the current GP workforce is too small to meet the demands of an expanding primary care service. The falling GP supply is compounded by the growing female practitioner workforce – their right to maternity leave, increasing trend towards part-time working and, as discussed earlier, a desire to retire early, which influence the supply side. One estimate is that 1.5 WTE GPs are needed to replace every leaver because of the tendency for recruits to work flexibly (Snell 2000a). Clearly, personnel issues are strongly tied to primary and community care workforce planning and development.

## Conclusion

Recruitment and retention cannot be ignored by managers as a result of the overlap between supply and demand for primary and community care staff and, therefore, they are another challenge facing personnel and general managers. An analysis of the literature showed that 85% of trust managers experience supply-side problems. Increasingly WP&D is a balance between the demand for staff and the supply of workers.

Today's recruitment and retention problems can easily upset primary and community workforce planning and development strategies. One in seven NHS workers is aged 50 years or older so the primary and community workforce is 'greying' and, worse, fewer younger people are being recruited. The greying phenomenon is affecting different sections of the workforce in dissimilar ways but practice nurses, as a professional group, are the oldest NHS workforce.

Moreover, the pool from which managers draw staff is shrinking and the public has a negative perception of the NHS as a career choice. Faced with problems such as these managers may not able to find the staff for their progressive and innovative workforce re-designs. NHS managers, on the other hand, have enjoyed major recruitment and retention success recently and the literature offers strong evidence on the ways they can capitalize on these successes (see Annotated bibliography, page 167).

Staff turnover in the NHS is higher than in the public sector generally. Losses vary among PCTs and between professional groups, but attrition is increasing uniformly in the NHS. The reasons why staff stay and leave are complex but rising workloads and unfilled vacancies are two of the most important in the list of factors that reduce job satisfaction at both ends of the age spectrum. Unfilled vacancies and continuing professional development failings, and administrative burden at the expense of clinical work also seem to have a disproportionate effect on a practitioner's desire to stay. Job satisfaction, about which there are comprehensive data from Healthcare Commission star-rating reviews, are given for each trust in the PCT WP&D database.

Some PCTs have eight times as many 3-month vacancies but rates vary remarkably. However, UK 'hotspots' are consistent and unsurprising because they are strongly associated with the housing market. Primary and community care professionals know they are in a 'seller's market' and can pick and choose where they work. Moreover, competition between the public and private sectors for health-care staff, especially AHPs, is increasing. The NHS Professionals scheme, although a stopgap solution to recruitment and retention problems, offers a cheaper option for managers than commercial agencies, and better employment conditions for participants.

Incidents of NHS workplace violence, approaching 100 000 per year, are a growing and emerging recruitment and retention problem. The PCT WP&D database shows that the number of crimes likely to affect primary and community care staff vary staggeringly between PCTs. This has major implications for all staff but especially out-of-hours practitioners. However, the literature offers sound guidance to help managers minimize the risks to isolated workers working in high crime areas (see Annotated bibliography, page 167).

*Improving Working Lives*, the Department of Health's recruitment and retention strategy, has been designed to diminish supply-side problems (NHS Executive 2000a). Consequently, PCT managers need to profile their workforce in a recruitment and retention context as well as reviewing the array of published guidance.

# CHAPTER EIGHT
# Determining team size and mix

## Demand-side methods

Ideally, primary and community workforce planning and development methods should be sensitive not only to community patient dependency and the workload generated but also to potential workload in the locality (Bowden 1987). However, Goldstone et al. (2000) suggest that most primary care trust (PCT) workforce planning systems are flawed not least because methods address only some of these issues, although managers have to use the best available information; in short, beggars can't be choosers. Other flaws in state-of-the-art primary and community care workforce planning include (Bowden 1987; Crawford et al. 1990; Audit Commission 1992a; Goodman 1996; Department of Health or DoH 2002b):

- ad hoc use and small gains seen as achievements
- irrational base data that are unconnected to best practice evidence
- poor information for evaluating workforce size and mix, especially a reliance on historical or retrospective data
- poor differentiation between health-care and social care dependency and workload
- unreliable or invalid recommendations caused by subjective interpretation of data coupled with processing errors
- budget rather than quality or equality driven.

Consequently, any workforce planning and development methods drawn from the community and primary care literature are going to be criticized. Therefore, triangulation (exploring the problem from different perspectives) should be used. As we have seen, many other workforce planning and development issues beset PCT managers, e.g. as a result of PCTs' different sizes and their special features, which makes each one unique, staffing formulae have to be standardized for manageability while still reflecting a PCT's unique features. One danger is that PCTs consistently at the 'undesirable end' of the morbidity, socioeconomic and other league tables would be unfairly assessed using, for example, the English average number of practitioners per head of population. Recommending an establishment for any PCT is unhelpful without understanding the morbidity, mortality and socioeconomic variables and related data. Banding similar PCTs is, therefore, one way of overcoming these problems and is a technique that shows great promise. Consequently, the Office for National Statistics (ONS) Bands, used extensively in the preceding chapters as a way of distinguishing between PCTs and their population demands, feature regularly in this chapter and the appendices.

Using data from PCTs that achieve better outcomes, such as longer life expectancy or higher Healthcare Commission (formerly the Commission for Health Improvement or CHI) star ratings, is another option explored in this chapter. Outcome data are improving in quantity and quality, and trust managers are much closer to knowing, other than by professional judgement, whether care standards are suffering as a consequence of poor staffing.

As discussed elsewhere, practitioners in some PCTs are twice as productive as their ONS Band counterparts. Any staffing recommendations, therefore, also need to equalize workloads for job satisfaction, recruitment and retention reasons. Consequently, these data feature heavily in the staffing algorithms used in this chapter and the appendices.

Another problem that PCT managers face is that nurse and health visitor staffing algorithms are unsuitable for therapists because the latter's workload could be driven by different variables such as referrals. Also, community and primary staff mix problems may need a solution that national databases cannot provide because health-care professionals in the Department of Health (DoH) databases are not broken down beyond:

- district nurses, health visitors and specialist practitioners (two staff groups)
- community staff nurses and school nurses (one homogeneous group)
- health-care assistants (one homogeneous group – who they support is unknown)
- GPs, practice nurses and nurse practitioners (two groups)
- administrative staff (one homogeneous group)
- allied health professionals (four groups).

This is a particularly frustrating issue for PCT managers. Unfortunately, the problems do not end here, i.e. the literature does not recommend appropriate numerators and denominators (explored later). The final problem, one that is only just emerging, is that modern primary and community care workforce planning is based on *Liberating the Talents* (DoH 2002c) and Evercare staffing labels, which are not supported by empirically determined data. At best, managers can rely only on professional judgement – one of the weakest workforce planning methods.

Probably as a consequence of these flaws and unknowns, evidence from the literature and national databases highlights several methods and data sources for estimating the number (and mix) of staff needed to meet primary and community workloads. Methods in the literature can be placed into four broad categories:

1. Professional judgement or consensus approaches
2. Population health needs based
3. Caseload analysis
4. Acuity or workload methods that use patient dependency classification and activity times.

# Professional judgement

The first broad method, professionally judging the level of staffing with safety and quality in mind, is identical to the inpatient counterpart of the same name (Waite 1986; Goldstone et al. 2000). A team of locally knowledgeable managers and practitioners decides the size and mix of teams for specific locations. This method is quick and inexpensive even though users often consider the following comprehensive list of variables and related data, but only in a broad, descriptive way (Bowden 1987; Crawford et al. 1990; Audit Commission 1992a, 1999; Lightfoot 1993; Seymour 1994; Prideaux 1996; Rink et al. 1996; DoH 2002b, 2002c):

• social care and health-care issues
• caseload profiles and existing practitioner records
• local health and school plans
• current team size and mix, which is usually historically based
• budget constraints and freedoms
• practitioner:population ratios
• service priorities and staff shortages
• job descriptions, practitioner roles and competencies
• emerging policies such as *Liberating the Talents* and Modernisation Agency initiatives
• outputs and outcomes such as the quality of care
• population density and transport
• cross-boundary flow
• time out such as sickness absence
• recruitment and retention successes and failures
• impending retirements
• part-time:full-time staffing ratios
• supply-side data.

Critics question consultative methods because data in the list above are not always available and, bizarrely, teams of judges do not always include practitioners. Another important weakness is that the method is inflexible and insensitive to fluctuating workloads.

An example of professional judgement shows managers in one PCT in the author's fieldwork who carefully reviewed the team of therapists before recommending the changes in Table 8.1 designed to meet the growing demand in the community, GP referral and National Service Framework (NSF) expectations.

**Table 8.1** Changes designed to meet growing demands

| Grade | Inpatient area | Children's services | Dietetic service | Outreach team |
|---|---|---|---|---|
| Senior 1 therapist | | | | +2 |
| Senior 2 therapist | +2 | | | +1 |
| Senior 1 OT | | | | +2 |
| Senior 2 OT | | | | +1 |
| SaLT | +0.5 | +4 | | +1.5 |
| SaLT assistant | | +2.7 | | |
| NSF community dietitian | | | +3 | |
| NSF primary care dietitian | | | +2 | |
| Secondary care dietitian | | | +1 | |
| Coordinator | | | | +1 |
| Technical instructor | | | | +2 |
| Administrator | | | | +1 |

NSF, National Service Framework; OT, occupational therapist; SaLT, speech and language therapist.

Managers took care when considering demographic issues and policy developments before re-designing the therapy team.

## Population and health needs-based approaches

The second main workforce planning method uses demographic and biographical variables similar to the ones listed above. The difference here is that numerical data are used in the calculations rather than merely using locality data in a descriptive way (Coffey undated; Piggott 1988; Durrand 1989; Noakes and Johnson 1999; Ebeid 2000; DoH 2001a; Steele et al. 2001; Cochrane et al. 2002):

- population density, age profiles, growth and shrinkage – chosen for indicating the demand on services

- socioeconomic data such as deprivation, housing, low birthweights and deaths, which are good proxy indicators of community patient dependency
- morbidity and mortality data such as General Health Questionnaire (GHQ) scores, which are another proxy dependency measure
- Finished consultant episodes to help overcome urban–rural bias.

Most authors of the studies reviewed obtained these variables empirically and recently these data have been included in Department of Health and ONS databases. Consequently, each PCT's data have been summarized and can be downloaded from www.healthcareworkforce.org.uk.

Despite these valuable, centrally held data, Cochrane et al. (2002) found it necessary to synthesize proxy measures from multiple sources in their evaluation of primary and community health-care workforces. Rowe et al. (1995) used individual practitioner records as an additional source of medicosocial data, which when aggregated were used to deploy staff. However, as discussed in Chapter 3, practitioners' records can be narrative rather than numerically based, which makes aggregation difficult. Steele et al. (2001) add another caveat – the veracity of caseload data should be confirmed before they are used.

Once data anomalies have been ironed-out, Rowe et al. (1995) and Steele et al. (2001) believe that workforce planning based on an assessment of population needs is the preferred approach and certainly better than caseload-based methods. However, Bowden's (1987) review of the primary and community care literature showed that only 20% of workforce planners used population health needs analysis methods. This small percentage is odd because, if managers consider both met and unmet need in their communities, population- and health-based staffing algorithms and data provide a good base from which to determine the size and mix of the primary and community workforce (Bowden 1987; Elkan et al. 2000a; DoH 2002b).

One downside is that population and health needs information gathering by nurses adds to their non-productive work (Drennan 1990a), although data need not be collected solely by nurses, and information technology plays an important role. Also, and obviously, to make the population- and health needs-based method workable, staffing norms, such as the number of practitioners per head of population from more than one PCT, are required. However, as raised earlier, there is some debate about the right numerator – the population numerator can be either census data or GP list size. The latter, although more precise from a planning standpoint, may not cover the community population (Dalton et al. 1972), e.g. some health visitor staffing analyses in the literature were based on the number of mothers and babies registered with GPs (Hyatt 2003). However, localities have unregistered people such as homeless people and travellers (DoH 1993a). Similarly, using the right denominator is equally challenging, e.g. should the headcount, funded or actual whole-time equivalents (WTEs) be used (Dalton et al. 1972)? Without doubt, careful planning and execution are needed.

The Audit Commission (1999) and Dobby and Barnes (1987a) criticized crude practitioner:population ratios that do not account for age differences and other important variables in the population. However, the method's value lies in developing staffing algorithms that reflect a locality's deprivation or geographical spread (Steele et al. 2001). Despite these criticisms, managers have used practitioner:population ratios for several years.

## Health visitors

- The 1956 Jameson report recommended 1 health visitor per 4300 population (Bowden 1987) – a ratio that is similar to Rowe et al.'s (1995), i.e. 1:4683.
- Dalton et al. (1972) expressed their health visitor ratio differently: 1.5 (range 0.4–2.2) per 10 000 population.
- Burrell-Davies and Williams (1984) found similar health visitor ratios ranging from 1:3245 to 1:6234 depending on the locality (Bowden 1987).
- Bell and Moules (1985) estimated the ratio of health visitors to population as 1:4300. Their model, although outmoded, included important workload variables such as health-visiting activity for differently aged children.
- Klein and Tomlinson (1987a, 1987b) also adjusted their health-visiting formulae according to local conditions. Their ratios ranged from 0.14 to 0.3 WTE per 1000 population depending on deprivation in the area.
- The ratio of health visitors to families (rather than individuals) in the author's fieldwork ranged from 1:250 to 1:300.
- Crofts et al.'s (2000) study of health visitor:population ratios (1:5462), although historical, seemed rationally based on the population needs.
- Ledger (1987) felt that a realistic ratio in deprived areas was 1 WTE to 3000 people.

Managers can easily use these data for benchmarking purposes. Apart from inner city PCTs, health visitor establishments are less variable than indicated in the literature (Steele et al. 2001). Crofts et al. (2000) believe that child health surveillance data are an important planning component for the health visitor workforce and, in practice, an important driver, e.g. they estimate that a 10–20% increase in the number of income support claimants in a health visitor's caseload increases workload by 6% or around 100 contacts. Consequently, in this chapter the number of children aged 5 years and under is used as the numerator rather than the population.

Bowns et al. (2000), on the other hand, feel that the demand for health visiting services is falling and that it is possible to reduce services for low-risk families. However, radical service reductions such as these need careful monitoring especially if health visitors undertake more targeted public health work as advocated by *Liberating the Talents* (Steele et al. 2001).

### District nurses

Although the data are old, the Ministry of Health's 1.85 district nurses per 10 000 population ratio, rising to 2.5 in areas with a high proportion of elderly people, has a benchmarking value (Dalton et al. 1972).

The Audit Commission's (1999) data are illuminating. Not only were district nurse:population ratios provided but also standard deviations. The mean was 8:10 000 population (SD = 15.4, $n$ = 43), which shows how skewed these data are. Indeed, the PCT workforce planning and development (WP&D) database analysed throughout this book shows trusts of similar size employing grossly different numbers of district nurses, leading the author to conclude that primary and community workforce planning is irrational.

The PCTs with proportionally older people in their population have intermediate care and intensive home support scheme issues, which means that the district nursing workforce needs special attention and consideration. Free nursing home care demands could easily counterbalance population effects, whereas chronic disease management and pastoral care are likely to shift staff mix towards health-care assistants. NSFs are likely to place extra demands on the community and primary care workforce, e.g. the Older Person's NSF asks workforce planners to create local workforces designed for older populations. It is anticipated that a third of the extra 20 000 nurses and 6500 therapists discussed in *The NHS Plan* are destined to care for elderly people (DoH 2002g). How staff mix is decided is not explained, but this chapter will help.

Morbidity and mortality data (see Chapter 3) offer plenty of scope for planning and developing the workforce with a growing preventive healthcare role. If, as *Liberating the Talents* (DoH 2002c) suggests, prevention increasingly falls into the remit of the community practitioner workforce, then both size and mix will need adjusting to accommodate a health prevention approach. These changes have workforce development, notably educational, implications too.

The case study PCT, used throughout the preceding chapters, is in the top 10% of high crime areas. This not only has quality-of-life implications for the population but also job safety issues for the workforce who work alone and are potentially vulnerable. Consideration has to be given to doubling up staff in high crime areas and providing mobile phones and personal alarms, particularly if a largely female workforce undertake more out-of-hours duties. These issues have been explored in more detail in Chapter 7.

## School nurses

- Lochead (1994) estimated an equitable ratio for school nurses at 1:3000–4000 population plus one assistant to four school nurses.
- The Court report (Bowden 1987) recommended a lower school nurse ratio of 1 nurse to 2500 school children.
- Whitmore et al.'s (1982a) ratios, although dated, ranged from 1 WTE to 401 pupils to 1:2135. Unsurprisingly, contact time varied as widely.
- Whyte's (1984) dated study based school nurse staffing on the number of annual health checks and concluded a ratio of one nurse to 2400 pupils. Health-care assistant support is also discussed but ratios or proportions are not given.

## Practice nurses

Practice nurses are the fastest growing group of health-care professionals. However, growth seems more reactive than planned:

- Hirst et al. (1998) noted that the GP:practice nurse ratio was uniform and that the best dependent variables for estimating practice nurse numbers were population and practice characteristics (a technique used later in this chapter). Although numbers are growing, there were still geographical disparities and the inverse care law applied. Raising practice nurse establishments to the best meant a 2100 WTE increase in the whole NHS workforce. Without these increases, workload equity becomes a serious issue.
- Bowling's (1987) ratio was 1:24 703 (SD = 12 900).
- Obeid (1997) felt that 0.25 WTE to 1000 patients was the minimum ratio. Establishments below this meant that practitioners struggled with their workloads.

The number of practice nurses in the UK grew irrationally by 73% in the 1990s (Audit Commission 1992a, 1999), which may be one reason why some PCTs in the WP&D database are practice nurse rich. However, these staff may be compensating for the lack of GPs, which is borne out by the above-average access and immunization performance data, i.e. access to GPs within 48 hours in our case study PCT is in the top 15%. If practice nurses are contributing to this above-average performance, then investment in them may pay dividends. Confusingly, however, patient access to other primary care practitioners, including practice nurses, is below average. Practice nurse-rich workforces are well placed to meet the demands of the new General Medical Service (GMS) contract, so creation of better access for patients using practice nurse- and nurse practitioner-led services is a strong possibility in many PCTs.

Populations served by these primary care practitioners are growing and ageing whereas the public's expectations are rising. Managers in PCTs that are GP poor, such as our case study PCT, also need to pay attention to workforce structure, e.g. as raised in Chapter 7 more women and part-time workers are joining whereas the average GP age is increasing; maternity leave is more common and the number retiring early is growing. Consequently, the UK long-term GP vacancy rate is 8%. Not only have practice managers found it increasingly hard to recruit GPs but also many clinicians are broadening their administrative and managerial duties, including PCT-related duties at the expense of clinical work (Goldacre 1998; DoH 2000a; Medical Practices Committee or MPC 2001). Developments such as the walk-in centres, expanding nursing roles and improving health in the population, on the other hand, could reduce service demand. Also, rising costs may force PCT managers to look for cheaper alternatives (Goldacre 1998; DoH 2000a).

Clearly, practitioner:population ratios should not be static but Rookes (1982) criticizes the inflexibility of some staffing ratios. Burrell-Davies and Williams (1984), on the other hand, showed improving ratios for the 3 years from 1979 to 1981. The health visitor staffing:population ratio in one region improved from 1:5271 (SD = 672) to 1:4995 (SD = 821). However, the ratios of other professionals, such as school nurses in the same locality, were not provided and data are needed to see whether staffing improvements are consistent. These worries are not unfounded because the author's fieldwork showed the irrationality of actual workforces. The PCT staff mix varied not only between ONS bands but also between PCTs in the same band. Steele et al. (2001) also noted little relationship between population need and staff number/mix. One implication of the more equitable staffing arising from ONS and workload-based ratios discussed later is that PCT managers will experience major increases or decreases, up to a third in some cases. Diversion of practitioners from over-staffed to under-staffed areas, even within the same PCT, is likely to be resisted (Steele et al. 2001).

## Caseload-based methods

The third broad workforce planning method, caseload analysis, which includes data such as the number of contacts, is another important and useful PCT workforce planning method (Waite 1986; Luft 1990; Frame and O'Donnell 1996). Bowden (1987) reported that this method was used by 23% of her respondents. Caseloads are determined by the community's needs so practitioners' caseload is potentially the size of the GP list (DoH 1993a).

However, Drennan (1990b) showed that similar-sized caseloads did not always generate the same amount of work, i.e. caseload size did not always equate to workload. This issue is important because Buchan (1999) explains how stress-related job dissatisfaction is influenced by workload; therefore, caseload data are also recruitment and retention variables. Authors such as the Audit Commission (1999), Barret and Hudson (1997), Dewis (2001), and Dobby and Barnes (1987a) indicate the information needed for caseload analysis although information will vary depending on the professional group being studied:

- service objectives and referral criteria
- new referrals
- patients' age distribution
- number and type of assessments and reassessments
- essential and non-essential activity
- direct and indirect care levels
- clerical and administrative work levels
- travelling time
- length of time the patient has spent on the practitioners' caseload.

Dewis (2001) and Frame and O'Donnell (1996) recommend that model caseloads be built from these data and that practice teams be benchmarked against them – a technique that is explained later. Outcomes alert managers to unfair workloads, which provide arguments for more or fewer resources. In short, these data are invaluable not only for modifying practitioners' workload and establishing equity, but also to review the number and mix of staff.

However, there is plenty of warning in the literature about using data such as the number of contacts solely to estimate staffing levels (Audit Commission 1992a, 1999; Heath 1994; Seymour 1994; Richards et al. 2000), e.g. activity data quickly become outmoded and need to be refreshed periodically. Unlike the ones used later, not all caseload methods have algorithms that are sensitive to demographic, socioeconomic, morbidity and mortality differences. Managers therefore need to take care about which benchmarks are used (Rookes 1982; Klein and Tomlinson 1987a, 1987b; Audit Commission 1992a; Heath 1994; Frame and O'Donnell 1996; Prideaux 1996; Dewis 2001).

Authors also criticize these methods because some exclude an overhead (e.g. administrative work) and time out and, more importantly, attempt to reduce community nursing to a list of mechanistic tasks.

Nevertheless, Crofts et al. (2000) feel that thoughtful application of these methods is critical, e.g. focusing on health visitor caseloads generally is likely to lead to staffing reductions when proportionally greater numbers of child protection cases will reverse the trend.

When these data and methods are applied they can be particularly useful in specific situations. From data collected by the author it is clear that some PCTs were considerably better staffed than either the England or their ONS Band average, e.g. the relationship between the number of therapists and the population size was statistically significant ($r_s$ = 0.31, $p$ = 0.001). However, therapists in some PCTs were considerably more productive than either the England or Band average. One explanation is that GPs in the author's fieldwork sites (who were grossly under-staffed in comparison to similar PCTs) were referring more cases, which may explain these differences. Clearly, something is driving demand for therapy services, which probably lies not only in staffing shortfalls in some professional groups but also the adverse morbidity and socioeconomic data discussed earlier. Physiotherapists in one of the author's fieldwork sites saw 15 new patients, whereas the professional body's recommendation was 10 new patients per week. Managers, however, felt that 12 patients per week was a more realistic figure considering the rising demand and staff shortages. Clearly, allied health professional (AHP) workloads in these PCTs would be unacceptable were they staffed as a 'typical' trust. The activity data summarized later throw considerable light on the difference between local and national AHP benchmarks and their implications.

Careful caseload analysis explained the reason for seemingly underperforming health visitors in one fieldwork site – the disproportionate number of child protection registrations and lone parents in the area. Conversely, the PCT study site district nurses were more productive, not only more than the England average but also up to twice the rate of the ONS Band average. However, although staff should be commended, PCT managers will have to consider whether this workload is equitable and sustainable. Barret and Hudson (1997) showed that the numbers of home visits are falling but each visit lasted longer. Increasingly, more time is being spent on technical care and patient education, whereas basic care time fell (probably caused by growing Social Service involvement). One implication is that number of contacts alone may not be an appropriate workload indicator unless related data are carefully considered.

# Dependency–acuity approaches

There is an overlap between the caseload analysis approach and the fourth, broad workforce-planning category – the dependency–acuity method – although this uses more generalized data (Audit Commission 1999). Goldstone et al. (2000) developed and tested the dependency–acuity method extensively in the community, the work he and his colleagues began 25 years earlier (Goldstone and Worrall 1980). The authors conclude that data collected systematically help primary and community workforce planners

(Goldstone et al. 2000, p. 39); examples are:

- patient characteristics including dependency and weighting indicating the level of family support
- staff activity such as professionally determined timings for patients in each dependency category
- workload indices
- quality of care
- staff absence and turnover

The dependency–acuity protocol is clear and logical:

- Each patient is assigned to a dependency group ranging from 1 (minimum care) to 4 (maximum) using a simple, activities-of-living rating scale.
- To accommodate domestic variables, weightings are included in the patient's dependency score:
  - below-average family support
  - average family support.

Dependency and the corresponding amount of nursing effort (in minutes) are entered into a simple algorithm given in Goldstone et al. (2000).

Similarly, Rookes (1982) devised a points system that indicates light-to-heavy health-visiting workloads:

- children under 5 years
- dependent families
- over-65s
- physically and mentally disabled individuals
- practice list size
- number of clinics
- day nursery and child-minder visits
- fieldwork teacher responsibilities.

Four outcomes emerged:

1. A workload factor for each health visitor
2. Separate clinic workload indicators
3. Group workload index
4. Percentage of time spent on key activities.

Rookes' article also includes a simple algorithm that converts these into ideal staff numbers. Prideaux (1996) devised a workload measure from not only the number and length of contacts but also the interventions involved. Moreover, Prideaux (1996) overcame the overhead criticism noted above by adding an indirect care and associated work component.

Rink et al. (1996) asked staff to complete activity diaries at 15-minute intervals coupled with daily reflection on the day's work for 1 week. Interestingly, these authors were some of the few researchers to include care quality measures in their fieldwork. Consequently, acuity, personal reflection and patient satisfaction were triangulated to provide a reasonably complete picture of appropriate and inappropriate working.

The advantage of community dependency–acuity systems is that they offer a standardized approach that avoids duplication and allows data aggregation. The validity and reliability of instruments can easily be tested (compared with, for example, health needs assessment). With attention, these methods accommodate overheads such as travelling time more easily than the other three approaches (Goldstone et al. 2000; Steele et al. 2001). Unlike hospitals the community is never 'full', which makes workload measures even more important. Consequently, primary and community care dependency–acuity data have several valuable functions (Coffey, undated; Fitton 1984b; Luft 1990; Frame and O'Donnell 1996):

• Using the number and length of practitioner–patient contacts to generate forecast hours, which are compared with available hours. A 10% difference between available and forecast hours is deemed tolerable.
• Tracking and comparing dependency and workload not only over time but also between areas and a means of checking equity, its effect on job satisfaction, recruitment and retention.
• Not only equalizing but also rationalizing and prioritizing work.
• Highlighting mismatches between ideal and actual staffing.
• Indicating informal carers' contribution to patient care.
• Encouraging a common language between commissioners and practitioners.
• Assisting decision-making about the size and mix of community teams.
• Informing joint working with Social Services.

On the other hand, workload assessment methods are prone to false data reporting either deliberately or unconsciously, so independent checks are needed. Despite policing, dependency–acuity methods are accepted by practitioners probably as a result of bottom-up ownership (Goldstone et al. 2000; Steele et al. 2001). Attaching care times to dependency weightings may not, however, be enough (Coffey, undated). Drennan (1990a) explains how invaluable dependency and workload data can be but criticizes the method because inadequate staffing generates a workload index that perpetuates inadequate staffing. It is imperative, therefore, that a measure of the quality of care is included at the time of workload measurement (Dobby and Barnes 1987a). Another way of strengthening the dependency–acuity method is to combine the approach with another method such as staff:population ratios – the so-called 'workforce planning triangulation' (Hirst et al. 1998). It is this triangulation approach that is now adopted.

## Evaluating team size and mix

PCT managers are faced with three broad workforce planning and development questions and problems:

- Is the PCT's 'stock' of workers sufficient to meet the workload? Managers are usually faced with historically determined establishments that bear little relationship to the community's wants and needs. Consequently, practitioners continually question whether their workloads are equitable. If the size or mix or both is wrong then modernization of the workforce is a problem.
- Policy changes that aim to modernize the primary care workforce for doing things differently. Recently, *Liberating the Talents* (DoH 2002c) and Evercare's core functions encourage managers to develop an interdisciplinary workforce based on patient need. Unfortunately, as a result of meagre national data, these decisions have to be based on professional judgement for the foreseeable future.
- Developing knowledge and skills so that practitioners can work efficiently and effectively.

## Some algorithms

Adequate establishments and fair workloads preoccupy many PCT managers. As can be seen in the PCT WP&D database, the numbers of community practitioners per head of population fluctuate widely not only between ONS Bands but also between PCTs in the same Band. Readers are, therefore, forced to conclude that the size (and mix) of primary and community care teams is irrational. At best, establishments are historical and at worse they fail to meet local demands while generating inequitable workloads.

The NHS has increased its headcount of the nursing (+1.9%) and GP (+1.3%) workforce since 1999. However, evidence from the literature shows that staffing shortfalls persist, which are being corrected by overtime, bank and agency staff bought from existing resources or simply through staff goodwill. Authors acknowledge that establishments have grown but are being overtaken by patient demands, staff shortages and new policy developments such as the NSFs. Giving managers the tools and data to evaluate the size (and mix) of their teams has, therefore, never been more important. Unfortunately, PCT managers do not have the array of methods that are available to inpatient care managers. As we saw earlier, primary and community staff numbers and mix can be evaluated in four main ways (summarized earlier). But each is flawed and the results from one method are likely to be criticized by policy makers, managers and practitioners. Combining results from professional judgement and population ratio methods, for example, is remarkably robust and triangulating approaches give managers more confidence in their results. Unfortunately, results from these methods perpetuate the traditional workforce and have less value for an interdisciplinary and needs-led WP&D. At least, on the other hand, they will show whether PCT managers are comparatively well staffed or workloads are equitable.

There is an invaluable but bewildering number of centrally held databases from which to evaluate and adjust the PCT workforce. The Department of Health and ONS databases hold workforce planning-related variables and data that are easily accessible and usable. But there are traps, e.g. using national population ratio averages for evaluating the PCT workforce leads to inappropriate results because of the different PCT characteristics. Consequently, the Healthcare Commission star rating and other information, aligned to ONS-banded PCTs in the database, allow managers to extrapolate from best practice and similar ONS trusts. Managers should, therefore, use data drawn only from areas that are demographically, socioeconomically similar to their own with similar morbidity data.

Other important considerations, as we saw earlier, include which denominators and numerators are used for staffing ratios, e.g. is the PCT population or GP list size the best numerator? For health visitors, should the PCT population or the number of children under 6 years be used? For the denominator, is the funded, actual or headcount establishment the best? Fortunately, the PCT WP&D database and algorithms provided have maximum flexibility, and the data have been standardized after considering the options.

As explored earlier, caseload profiling, notably the number of patient contacts per practitioner, is one way of estimating workforce size. A major feature of the PCT WP&D database is contacts per practitioner from 'best-practice' PCTs and also trusts from the same ONS Band. These data are excellent for equalizing workloads – an important job satisfaction, recruitment and retention issue. Although the literature regularly questions the veracity of these data, secondary analysis of the PCT WP&D database indicates that activity data may be more robust than thought, e.g. the size of the workforce (in WTEs) is strongly correlated to the number of contacts that practitioners generate. In short, the PCT WP&D database is recommended.

In the tables in the appendices, morbidity, mortality, socioeconomic and performance data from a second case study PCT are consolidated. After reading the tables and commentaries, the reader is encouraged to download his or her or PCT's data from www.healthcareworkforce.org.uk and replace the specimen PCT's data with his or her trust's values. Reviewing the commentaries in the light of the new data will help to consolidate the main workforce planning and development issues. The variables in the tables are defined in the PCT WP&D database.

## Modernizing the PCT workforce

One main problem persists, however. Existing variables and data are based on traditional workforces. New health policies such as the new GMS contract, *Liberating the Talents* and Evercare make these formulae and algorithms outmoded. Unfortunately, there are no or very few databases to help PCT managers reconfigure traditional workforces along the traditional lines of *Liberating the Talents*. Nevertheless, the downloadable PCT WP&D database generates considerable insight into the probable new primary and community care roles. After reviewing this and Chapter 7, questions that PCT managers might ask include:

- What are the local morbidity, mortality and socioeconomic issues and do these suggest a certain staff mix?
- Specifically, what are the first contact, chronic disease management and public health issues?
- How do local staff ratios compare with PCT staff ratios in the same ONS Band and also with three-star PCTs? Is any staff group establishment particularly better or worse off?
- Is the relationship between the staffing and activity (number of contacts) significant? For example, are understaffed groups also highly productive and vice versa?
- What is the ratio of registered practitioners to health-care assistants? If the workforce is reliant on assistants, are qualified staff acting in a more supervisory role?

# Demographic data

Rows and columns, which are inversed, equate to the PCT WP&D database www.healthcarework-force.org.uk (where variables are defined).

| Column | Row Variable | 7 England average | 21 Three-star PCTs | 12 ONS 1 | 13 ONS 2 | 14 ONS 3 | 15 ONS 4 | 16 ONS 5 | 17 ONS 6 | Specimen PCT | PCT's per-centile |
|---|---|---|---|---|---|---|---|---|---|---|---|
| F | ONS Band | | | | | | | | | 6 | |
| G | PCT population | 153 430 | 147 977 | 204 105 | 143 541 | 160 279 | 154 343 | 159 510 | 140 910 | 272 465 | 95th |
| I | GP list size | 155 131 | 149 683 | 250 883 | 154 805 | 155 042 | 168 712 | 170 439 | 144 778 | 280 633 | 95th |
| K | Females (%) | 51.3 | 51.4 | 51.8 | 51.5 | 51.4 | 51.7 | 51.1 | 51.2 | 51.6 | 70th |
| L | < 6 years (%) | 5.9 | 5.6 | 6.6 | 5.8 | 6.1 | 5.7 | 6.1 | 5.5 | 5.3 | 20th |
| M | 6–15 years (%) | 14.3 | 14.4 | 12.2 | 14.7 | 14.8 | 13.9 | 14.3 | 13.9 | 13.3 | 18th |
| N | 16–24 years (%) | 10 | 9.8 | 12.8 | 10.2 | 11.1 | 10.4 | 9.7 | 9.6 | 11.8 | 77th |
| O | 25–64 years (%) | 53.2 | 53 | 58.5 | 52.7 | 51.8 | 53 | 54.0 | 53.1 | 53.4 | 50th |
| P | > 64 years (%) | 16 | 16.3 | 10.4 | 15.7 | 15.6 | 16.5 | 15.0 | 16.9 | 16.3 | 55th |
| Q | Mean age (years) | 38.8 | 39.4 | 34.7 | 38.7 | 37.9 | 39 | 38.4 | 39.8 | 39.3 | 60th |
| R | Population growth (%) | 0.15 | 0.08 | 0.63 | 0.06 | 0.15 | 0.12 | 0.31 | 0.03 | 0.04 | 35th |
| S | Population density | 2427 | 1932 | 11 247 | 3980 | 5987 | 2687 | 1828 | 1224 | 1240 | 31st |
| AV | Without a car (%) | 24 | 22 | 54 | 33 | 32 | 24.5 | 18 | 22 | 24 | 50th |
| T | Ethnicity (white %) | 93.4 | 96 | 52.5 | 96.5 | 86.9 | 93.5 | 91.7 | 96.6 | 96.7 | 79th |

## Commentary

| Column | Profile issue (column items relate to those above) | Workforce planning and development implications |
|---|---|---|
| G I | Large PCT but more patients are registered with GPs than the census population indicates (university city) | PCT staffing calculations based on census populations may be inequitable |
| K | More females | Will recruitment be easier locally? |
| L to N | Fewer toddlers and teenagers but population is growing. More young adults because the PCT sits in a university city | Is there scope for health promotion? Boost public health roles? |
| P | Average elderly population | Less demand for chronic disease management? |
| S, AV | Low population density and average car ownership | Longer practitioner travelling time so establish satellite clinics and geographic working? |

# APPENDIX II

# Socioeconomic and health needs assessment

Rows and columns, which are inversed, equate to the database.

| Column | Row<br>Variable | 7<br>England<br>average | 21<br>Three-star<br>PCTs | 12<br>ONS 1 | 13<br>ONS 2 | 14<br>ONS 3 | 15<br>ONS 4 | 16<br>ONS 5 | 17<br>ONS 6 | Specimen<br>PCT | PCT's<br>per-<br>centile |
|---|---|---|---|---|---|---|---|---|---|---|---|
| F | ONS Band | | | | | | | | | 6 | |
| U | Acutely ill (%) | 15.1 | 14.8 | 18.6 | 17.5 | 14.3 | 15.2 | 14.3 | 14.4 | 13.2 | 18th |
| V | GHQ ill-health (%) | 16.8 | 16.3 | 22.1 | 17.6 | 16.3 | 18.6 | 17.5 | 15.7 | 13.6 | 15th |
| W | Fair to bad health (%) | 23.8 | 24.5 | 27.8 | 30.5 | 27.2 | 22.9 | 19.2 | 24.1 | 21.6 | 33rd |
| X | Poor general health (%) | 8.9 | 8.8 | 8.6 | 11.8 | 10.1 | 8.7 | 6.9 | 9.4 | 7.9 | 35th |
| Y | Young chronically ill(%) | 13.0 | 13.1 | 12.5 | 17.4 | 14.3 | 12.7 | 10.2 | 14.1 | 11.1 | 28th |
| Z | Chronically ill (%) | 17.9 | 18.3 | 15.6 | 21.8 | 18.6 | 17.4 | 14.6 | 19.0 | 16.4 | 35th |
| AA | Permanently sick (%) | 4.8 | 4.9 | 5.1 | 8.4 | 6.1 | 4.7 | 3.2 | 5.3 | 3.8 | 28th |
| AB | Disability claimants (%) | 6.2 | 6.6 | 5.0 | 8.9 | 6.8 | 5.8 | 4.4 | 6.7 | 4.7 | 48th |
| AC | Daily cigarettes | 4.0 | 3.8 | 4.7 | 5.0 | 4.1 | 3.9 | 3.6 | 3.7 | 3.6 | 30th |
| AD | Wheezers (%) | 33.5 | 34.7 | 37.8 | 34.6 | 33.3 | 35.8 | 31.8 | 32.7 | 31.1 | 25th |
| AE | BMI > 30 (%) | 17.0 | 17.9 | 14.2 | 17.8 | 17.8 | 15.8 | 15.6 | 18.1 | 16.3 | 38th |
| AF | Alcohol > 35 units (%) | 4.2 | 4.2 | 5.6 | 5.2 | 5.1 | 3.5 | 4.1 | 3.9 | 4.2 | 50th |
| AG | Accidents to hospital (%) | 18.2 | 18.8 | 13.0 | 19.0 | 18.6 | 18.3 | 18.2 | 17.2 | 17.9 | 45th |
| BL | Population FCE ratio | 4.5 | 4.5 | 5.7 | 3.7 | 4.4 | 4.5 | 5.5 | 4.3 | 5.0 | 67th |
| AH | Prescribed medication (%) | 42.7 | 45.1 | 39.1 | 45.1 | 42.1 | 42.7 | 41.1 | 43.3 | 42.0 | 45th |
| AI | Band A housing (%) | 19.7 | 23 | 2.2 | 58.3 | 42.0 | 10.3 | 6.9 | 30.9 | 19.1 | 45th |
| AJ | No central heating/bath (%) | 0.09 | 0.07 | 0.61 | 0.05 | 0.13 | 0.18 | 0.07 | 0.08 | 0.10 | 53rd |
| AK | ≥ first floor and above accommodation (%) | 7.8 | 6.3 | 44.9 | 6.1 | 9.2 | 11.6 | 8.7 | 5.9 | 6.2 | 32nd |
| AL | Lone parent and child (%) | 5.8 | 5.7 | 8.2 | 7.4 | 7.5 | 6.1 | 5.0 | 5.5 | 5.1 | 30th |
| AM | Child protection registration (%) | 0.047 | 0.05 | 0.070 | 0.052 | 0.021 | 0.05 | 0.045 | 0.062 | 0.013 | 5th |
| AN | Lone pensioner (%) | 14.4 | 14.4 | 11.6 | 15.1 | 14.8 | 14.3 | 13.4 | 14.6 | 14.4 | 50th |
| AO | Unpaid carer > 50 h (%) | 20.0 | 19.3 | 19.5 | 24.4 | 21.7 | 19.7 | 16.7 | 20.7 | 17.8 | 30th |
| AP | Home care (hours per capita) | 0.053 | 0.05 | 0.085 | 0.061 | 0.019 | 0.05 | 0.050 | 0.056 | 0.013 | 5th |
| AQ | Care home population (%) | 0.56 | 0.66 | 0.13 | 0.59 | 0.46 | 0.7 | 0.51 | 0.62 | 0.53 | 45th |
| AR | Crime rate per 1000 population | 44 | 40 | 102 | 55 | 72 | 39 | 33 | 37 | 39 | 45th |
| AS | Unemployed (%) | 3.0 | 3 | 5.7 | 4.1 | 3.8 | 3.1 | 2.3 | 3.0 | 2.4 | 30th |
| AT | Deprivation rank ($n = 354$) | 144 | 166 | 26 | 42 | 92 | 133 | 268 | 143 | 226 | 72nd |
| AV | Without a car (%) | 24 | 22 | 54 | 33 | 32 | 24.5 | 18 | 22 | 24 | 50th |

FCE, finished consultant episode; GHQ, General Health Questionnaire.

# Commentary

| Column | Profile issue (column items relate to those above) | Workforce planning and development implications |
|---|---|---|
| U | Lower levels of work-preventing acute illness | Primary and community care staff time out may also be lower |
| AG, BL | Low finished consultant episode per capita but more accidents requiring hospital treatment | Equivocal demand for technical care in the community<br>Scope for health promotion |
| V, AB | Consistently low levels of chronic illness but more in the young than ONS 6 (but still low) | Less demand for chronic disease management workers?<br>Staff mix needs to be health-care assistant rich? |
| AC, AF | Low smoking and average alcohol intake | May influence the PCT's health promotion strategy |
| AI<br>AT | Smaller proportion of Band A houses<br>Affluent area with pockets of deprivation | Raises health equality issues, which has implications for meeting the needs of the under-served |
| AM | Child protection registrants virtually non-existent | Implications for health visitors and social services |
| AR | Above average person/property crime rate | Out-of-hours worker safety, which may call for pairing staff working in high-risk areas |
| P, AN, AP, AQ | Fewer older people<br>Average number of lone pensioners<br>Negligible Social Service home care<br>Smaller care home population | Equivocal care of the elderly issues<br>Government's 'free care home nursing' policy implications |

## Appendix III

# Staff activity and evaluating team size

Columns and rows, which are inversed, equate to the PCT WP&D database.

| Column | Row Variable | 7 England average | 21 Three-star PCTs | 12 ONS 1 | 13 ONS 2 | 14 ONS 3 | 15 ONS 4 | 16 ONS 5 | 17 ONS 6 | Specimen PCT | PCT's per-centile |
|---|---|---|---|---|---|---|---|---|---|---|---|
| F | ONS Band | | | | | | | | | 6 | |
| BY | HV < 6-year PR | 306 | 278 | 354 | 261 | 308 | 302 | 331 | 302 | 243 | 24th |
| BZ | HV PR | 5346 | 4955 | 5020 | 4759 | 5229 | 5705 | 5413 | 5327 | 4628 | 28th |
| CA | DN PR | 5059 | 5131 | 5632 | 4573 | 6886 | 5324 | 5078 | 4901 | 11780 | 98th |
| CB | Community SN PR | 2952 | 2429 | 2576 | 2340 | 2362 | 3183 | 4042 | 2965 | 2399 | 35th |
| CC | HCA PR | 3986 | 4129 | 4055 | 5124 | 5428 | 3006 | 3960 | 3240 | 1756 | 18th |
| CD | GP PR | 1742 | 1732 | 1683 | 1972 | 1828 | 1711 | 1711 | 1678 | 1458 | 8th |
| CE | GP list size ratio | 2009 | 1932 | 2136 | 1981 | 2015 | 2040 | 1968 | 1954 | 1725 | 8th |
| CF | PN PR | 4582 | 4509 | 4889 | 4467 | 4375 | 4845 | 4797 | 4437 | 4429 | 40th |
| CG | GP admin PR | 999 | 989 | 984 | 928 | 987 | 1019 | 1046 | 999 | 1144 | 91st |
| CH | Podiatrist PR | 13 466 | 11 401 | 14 931 | 10 494 | 14 159 | 14 030 | 14 999 | 13 473 | 12 126 | 45th |
| CI | Dietitian PR | 31 927 | 22 210 | 92 445 | 17 655 | 41 352 | 26 769 | 32 518 | 31 154 | NA | |
| CJ | OT PR | 12 166 | 8377 | 15 242 | 14 597 | 25 089 | 10 050 | 13 586 | 9109 | 3310 | 7th |
| CK | PT PR | 9485 | 7687 | 21 323 | 8876 | 15 929 | 8309 | 8587 | 8725 | NA | |
| CL | SaLT PR | 9609 | 10 911 | 10 253 | 9743 | 9272 | 9560 | 9149 | 11 479 | 13 596 | 65th |
| CM | HV/DN vacancies (%) | 1.6 | 1.33 | 6.42 | 1.3 | 1.3 | 2 | 2.23 | 1.33 | 0.97 | 20th |
| CN | AHP vacancies (%) | 4.2 | 3.9 | 6.7 | 4.1 | 5.1 | 5.9 | 4.7 | 3.8 | 3.0 | 10th |
| CO | Full/part-time ratio | 1.39 | 1.42 | 1.33 | 1.34 | 1.34 | 1.34 | 1.46 | 1.39 | 1.48 | 90th |
| CP | Sickness absence (%) | 4.1 | 4 | 4.5 | 4.3 | 4.1 | 4.2 | 3.7 | 4.2 | 3.4 | 30th |
| BF | HV contact ratio | 1356 | 1193 | 1185 | 1553 | 1055 | 1535 | 1580 | 1234 | 1009 | 26th |
| BG | DN contact ratio | 395 | 405 | 354 | 648 | 783 | 365 | 310 | 451 | 801 | 78th |
| BH | Podiatrist contact ratio | 1034 | 937 | 687 | 921 | 1156 | 967 | 1127 | 1067 | 698 | 16th |
| BI | OT contact ratio | 83 | 112 | | 85 | 131 | 79 | 79 | 103 | 96 | 55th |
| BJ | PT contact ratio | 296 | 337 | 296 | 217 | 244 | 334 | 290 | 330 | NA | |
| BS | Staff satisfaction (Likert) | 3 | 3 | 2.8 | 3 | 3 | 3 | 3 | 3 | 3 | 50th |

DN, district nurse; HV, health visitor; OT, occupational therapist; PN, practice nurse; PR, population ratio; PT, physiotherapist; SaLT, speech and language therapist; SN, community staff nurse.

## Commentary

| Column | Profile issue (column items relate to those above) | Workforce planning and development implications |
|---|---|---|
| BY, BF | 24% more health visitors, who are 18% less productive | Boost health visitor public health and chronic disease management roles? |
| CA | 58% fewer district nurses, who are 44% more productive (one of the smallest district nursing workforces in England) | Implications for out-of-hours work? Supervision implications |
| CB | 19% more community staff nurses | Community staff nurses take on more chronic disease management roles and out-of-hours work? |
| CC | 46% more health-care assistants (HCAs). In the top 20% of HCA-rich workforces | Are district nurses working mainly as supervisors? |
| CD, CF | 13% more general practitioners (top 8%) Equitable practice nurse workforce | Meeting the demands of primary care first-contact work less of an issue? Scope for interdisciplinary care |
| CG | 13% fewer practice admin staff (bottom 10%) | Reduced scope for relieving practitioners' administrative burdens? |
| CH–CL | Mixed allied health professional (AHP) staffing but less productive | Boost allied health professionals' chronic disease management roles? |
| BS, CP, CM, CN | Employer satisfaction scores are high Below average sickness-absence levels Low vacancy rates | Recruitment and retention seems to be less of an issue for the PCT |

# Appendix IV
# Efficiency and effectiveness

Rows and columns, which are inversed, equate to the PCT WP&D database.

| Column | Row Variable | 7 England average | 21 Three-star PCTs | 12 ONS 1 | 13 ONS 2 | 14 ONS 3 | 15 ONS 4 | 16 ONS 5 | 17 ONS 6 | Specimen PCT | PCT's per-centile |
|---|---|---|---|---|---|---|---|---|---|---|---|
| F | ONS Band | | | | | | | | | 6 | |
| AW | CHI stars | 2 | 3 | 1 | 2 | 2 | 2 | 2 | 2 | 3 | |
| AX | Male life expectancy | 75.5 | 75 | 74.6 | 73.6 | 74.3 | 75.7 | 76.5 | 76.5 | 75.6 | 70th |
| AY | Female life expectancy | 80.2 | 80.2 | 80.7 | 78.8 | 79.6 | 80.7 | 80.9 | 80.2 | 81.0 | 80th |
| AZ | CHD deaths per 100 000 | 118 | 123.7 | 125 | 150 | 129 | 110 | 104 | 119 | 110 | 38th |
| BA | Circulatory disease death improvement | 3 | 3 | 3 | 3 | 3 | 3 | 3 | 3 | 3 | |
| BB | Cancer death improvement | 3 | 3 | 3 | 3 | 3 | 3 | 3 | 3 | 3 | |
| BC | Breast cancer screening (%) | 78.4 | 80.8 | 54.5 | 78.6 | 76.2 | 76.1 | 77.9 | 81.1 | 83.0 | 88th |
| BD | Cervical/diabetic screening | 4.5 | 4.5 | 2.5 | 4.5 | 4.5 | 4.5 | 4.5 | 4.5 | 4.5 | |
| BE | Teenage pregnancy improvement | 3 | 4 | 3 | 4 | 3 | 3 | 3 | 3 | 3 | 30th |
| BK | Reference cost index | 113 | 102 | 147 | 101 | 114 | 112 | 123 | 109 | 124 | 61st |
| BLL | Population FCE ratio | 4.53 | 4.48 | 5.65 | 3.7 | 4.35 | 4.7 | 5.51 | 4.32 | 5.0 | 67th |
| BM | GP 48-h access | 2 | 2 | 2 | 2 | 2 | 2 | 2 | 2 | 2 | |
| BN | Access to nurse 24 h | 2 | 2 | 2 | 2 | 2 | 2 | 2 | 2 | 2 | |
| BO | 4-week smoke quitters | 2 | 2 | 2 | 2 | 2 | 2 | 2 | 2 | 2 | |
| BP | Delayed hospital transfer | 3 | 3 | 3 | 3 | 3 | 3 | 2 | 2 | 2 | 15th |
| BQ | Patient satisfaction | 3 | 3 | 3 | 3 | 3 | 3 | 3 | 3 | 3.2 | 95th |
| BR | Patient complaints per 10 000 population | 1.7 | 1.3 | 3.0 | 1.1 | 1.8 | 2.1 | 1.5 | 1.8 | 2.6 | 72nd |
| BT | CHD audit data < 1 year old (%) | 100.0 | 100.0 | 88.0 | 100.0 | 96.7 | 97.5 | 100.0 | 100.0 | 97.2 | 45th |
| BU | Timely equipment delivery | 3 | 3.5 | 3 | 3 | 3 | 3 | 3 | 3 | 3 | 30th |
| BV | Vaccination and immunization | 4 | 4 | 1 | 4 | 4 | 3.5 | 3.5 | 4 | 4 | 60th |

CHD, coronary heart disease; CHI, Commission for Health Improvement; FCE, finished consultant episode.

162

# Commentary

| Column | Profile issue (column items relate to those above) | Workforce planning and development implications |
|---|---|---|
| AZ–BB | Low tracer disease (e.g. coronary heart disease) mortality | |
| AX–AY | Longer life expectancy | |
| BC/D–BV | Good screening and immunization coverage | Capitalize on the practice nurses' performance |
| BE | Low but a lesser reduction in teenage pregnancies | Boost school public health practitioner role |
| BK | Higher reference cost index | Review staff number and mix |
| BL | Low FCE per capita | First contact implications |
| BM–BN | Good 24-/48-h access | Capitalize on the practice nurses' performance |
| BP | Greater delayed hospital transfer | Care home and intermediate care review needed? |
| BU | Delayed community equipment delivery | Implications for worker health and safety |
| BQ–BR | Good community patient satisfaction scores but more complaints | Tie complaints analysis with a staffing review? |

# Recruitment and retention

Row and columns, which are inversed, equate to the PCT WP&D database.

| Column | Row Variable | 7 England average | 21 Three-star PCTs | 12 ONS 1 | 13 ONS 2 | 14 ONS 3 | 15 ONS 4 | 16 ONS 5 | 17 ONS 6 | Specimen PCT | PCT's per-centile |
|---|---|---|---|---|---|---|---|---|---|---|---|
| F | ONS Band | | | | | | | | | 6 | |
| K | Females (%) | 51.3 | 51.4 | 51.8 | 51.5 | 51.4 | 51.7 | 51.1 | 51.2 | 51.6 | 70th |
| N | 16–24 years (%) | 10 | 9.8 | 12.8 | 10.2 | 11.1 | 10.4 | 9.7 | 9.6 | 11.8 | 77th |
| AU | No educational qualifications (%) | 29 | 28 | 22 | 35 | 32 | 27 | 24 | 31 | 26 | 31st |
| CM | HV/DN vacancies (%) | 1.6 | 1.3 | 6.4 | 1.3 | 1.3 | 2 | 2.2 | 1.3 | 1.0 | 20th |
| CN | AHP vacancies (%) | 4.2 | 3.9 | 6.7 | 4.1 | 5.1 | 5.9 | 4.7 | 3.8 | 3.0 | 10th |
| CO | Full:part time ratio | 1.39 | 1.42 | 1.33 | 1.34 | 1.34 | 1.37 | 1.46 | 1.39 | 1.48 | 90th |
| CP | Sick. absence (%) | 4.1 | 4 | 4.5 | 4.3 | 4.1 | 4.2 | 3.7 | 4.2 | 3.4 | 30th |
| BS | Staff satisfaction | 3 | 3 | 2.8 | 3 | 3 | 3 | 3 | 3 | 3 | 45th |
| CQ | Improving Working Lives | 2 | 2 | 2 | 2 | 2 | 2 | 2 | 2 | 2 | NA |

AHP, allied health professional; DN, district nurse; HV, health visitor.

## Commentary

| Column | Profile issue (column items relate to those above) | Workforce planning and development implications |
|---|---|---|
| K, AU, N | More females, above-average scholastic achievement<br>More young adults | NHS recruitment opportunities |
| CM, CN, CP | Low vacancy rates<br>Low sickness absence | Capitalize on the reasons why staff are more satisfied and take less sick leave |
| CO | More part-time workers | Job sharing, twilight shift work |
| CQ | Improving Working Lives | Met the target (as did the majority of other PCTs) |

# Annotated bibliography

It will help if the reader downloads the bibliography from www.healthcare-workforce.org.uk before turning on 'Document Map' or using Ctrl F to locate articles with specific key words such as 'dependency'.

ACPM/CSP. (2002) Recommendations for calculating physiotherapy staffing levels for GP referral musculoskeletal outpatient services. London: ACPM/CSP.

Provides useful benchmarks and algorithms for physiotherapy managers. Key words: staffing, activity.

Adams, E. (1997) Employment legislation for the UK: a European future? British Journal of Health Care Management 3: 492–498.

Looks at the employment-law implications of: parental leave; European Working Time Directive; sexual harassment; discrimination; minimum wage; and disputes. Key words: recruitment and retention, personnel.

Allen, C. (2001) Human resources: lean on me. Health Service Journal 111(5744): 32–33.

Provides valuable data and insight into the reduction of sickness absence, which workforce planners include in their staffing calculations. Addresses some aspects of *Improving Working Lives*. Key words: time out.

Almond, P. (2002) An analysis of the concept of equity and its application to health visiting. Journal of Advanced Nursing 37: 598–606.

Defines health-care equity and equality broadly and specifically for health visiting. Uses vignettes to explain both. The nature and value of health needs assessment are also covered as a means of directing health visiting. Adds to the public health role of health visiting in the context of *Liberating the Talents*. Describes seven measures of health visiting performance. Key words: staff activity, dependency, efficiency and effectiveness.

Anderson, W. (1991) Quality assurance in general practice. Medical Audit News 1(4): 50–51.

Simply and clearly explains clinical audit in general practice. While preferring the phrase 'clinical review', the author describes the strengths and weaknesses of three approaches: (1) practice activity analysis; (2) minimum standards of care; and (3) staff behaviour. Also recommends that GPs should act autonomously rather than having audit imposed. Key word: quality.

Andrews, K. (2004) Workforce Matters: Linking service need to workforce planning. London: DoH.

Discusses several primary and community care innovative work roles and related issues. Includes plenty of case studies and supporting data, which would be useful for *Liberating the Talents* workforce planning. Key words: staff mix.

Angel, S., Nicoll, J. and Amatiello, W. (1990) Assessing the need for an out-of-hours telephone advisory service. Health Visitor 63: 225–227.

Explains the need for and the potential value of an out-of-hours telephone advisory service run by health visitors. Key words: activity, first contact.

Anonymous (1994) IRS/RCN Survey: the impact of community care on district nurses. Occupational Health Review 52: 10–19.

Detailed empirical survey of community nurse working conditions after the early 1990s community reforms. Workload, work injury, stress, job satisfaction and care quality are considered. Organizationally dated but the principles survive. Key words: recruitment and retention.

Appleton, J.V. (1994) The role of the Health Visitor in identifying and working with vulnerable families in relation to child protection: a review of the literature. Journal of Advanced Nursing 20: 167–175.

Examines health visiting structures, processes and outcomes in the context of vulnerable families. Key words: staff activity.

Atkin, K. and Lunt, N. (1995) Nurses in Practice: The role of the practice nurse in primary health care. York University: Social Policy Research Unit.

Atkin, K. and Lunt, N. (1996) The role of the practice nurse in primary health care: managing and supervising the practice nurse resource. Journal of Nursing Management 4: 85–92.

Atkin, K., Lunt, N., Parker, M. et al. (1993) Nurses Count: A national census of practice nurse. York: York University, SPRU.

Atkin, K., Lunt, N. and Parker, M. (1994) The role and self-perceived training needs of nurses employed in general practice: observations from a national census of practice nurses in England and Wales. Journal of Advanced Nursing 20: 46–52.

Series of related articles and reports that examine the actual and likely trends of practice nurse structures, processes and outcome after the rapid growth in the number of practice nurses. Despite health-care professionals' resistance to change as a result of loss of autonomy, practice nurses were the most enthusiastic members of integrated teams. Takes GPs' and other practitioners' perspectives. Practice nurses' education and training issues are well covered. Key words: staff mix, staff activity, education and training.

Audit Commission (1986) Making a Reality of Community Care. London: Audit Commission.

Looks at the services offered to people in the community including joint working, efficiency and effectiveness. Key words: staff mix, cost and quality.

Audit Commission (1992a) Homeward Bound: A new course for community care. London: Audit Commission.

Although dated, explains the managerial and clinical implications of the purchaser–provider split. The arguments about efficiency and effectiveness are relevant today, however, particularly: the size and mix of nursing teams; clinical information systems; health needs analysis; staff activity; quality assurance; and joint working. Shows remarkable foresight about *Liberating the Talents* and clinical governance. Key words: dependency and acuity, staff mix, quality and cost, information management and technology.

Audit Commission (1992b) All in a Day's Work: An audit of day surgery in England and Wales. London: Audit Commission.

Looks at the community dependency and acuity implications of increasing day surgery. Key words: dependency and acuity.

Audit Commission (1994) Seen But Not Heard. London: HMSO

Detailed review leading to recommendations based on best practice for community child health services. Covers both NHS services and Social Services, individually and jointly. Useful data are provided; although out of date the principles apply. Key words: activity, staff mix, efficiency and effectiveness.

Audit Commission (1999) First Assessment. A review of district nursing services in England and Wales. London: Audit Commission.

Detailed examination of district nursing including: health needs; referrals; activity; service structure/process strength and weaknesses; practitioner likes and dislikes; and user views. Ample quantitative and qualitative data are provided and analysed. Before *Liberating the Talents* (LtT) but evidence can easily be extrapolated into the LtT framework. Key words: establishments, first contact, continuing care.

Barkauskas, V. (1983) Effectiveness of public health nurse home visits to primiparous mothers and their infants. American Journal of Public Health 73: 573–580.

Mothers' outcomes, using 13 variables, were compared with a cohort of women who had not had home contact with public health nurses. Only one variable was significant: health seeking behaviour by the intervention group. Author concludes that home visits are not as cost-effective and clinic or group activities could be substituted. Key words: activity, cost-effectiveness.

Barret, G. and Hudson, M. (1997) Changes in district nursing workload. Journal of Community Nursing 17(3): 4–8.

Examines the steady rise and implications in recent years of the number of referrals to district nurses. Compares and contrasts workload before and after the Community Care Act. Examines the staff-mix implications. Methods and data are given. Key word: acuity.

Barriball, L. and Mackenzie, A. (1993) Measuring the impact of nursing interventions in the community. Journal of Advanced Nursing 18: 401–407.

Reviews the literature relating to: community nursing health needs analysis; activity; effectiveness; outcomes; prevention; multidisciplinary interventions; and patient views and satisfaction. Organizationally outmoded but the principles apply. Key word: review.

Battle, S., Moran-Ellis, J. and Salter, B. (1985) Defining a role. Nursing Times Community Outlook 81: 41.

Organizationally dated but useful examination of district nursing activity based on a comprehensive review of care. Concludes that some personal care activities are inappropriately carried out by highly skilled district nurses. Key words: staff activity.

Bell, A. and Moules, E. (1985) Staffing levels. The demographic factor. Nursing Times 81(31): 28–30.

Uses activity analysis and population statistics to estimate health visitor workload and establishments. Structurally out of date but the principles apply. Key word: establishments.

Betts, G. (2003) Primary care: Home truths. Health Service Journal 113(5837): 26–27.

Anecdotal account of the quality and efficiency of elderly health and social care. Recommends strengthening elderly care in the community by creating a generic worker to span both domains. Key words: staff mix.

Billingham, K. (1991) Debate: Public health and the community health visitor. Health Visitor 64(2): 40–43.

Explains the development of health visitor roles into today's complex, multidimensional work. Argues that one professional cannot reasonably undertake the modern, complex role, which falls into three broad functions. Offers solutions for revising the health visitor's role. Key words: activity, staff mix.

Black, S. and Hagel, D. (1996) Developing and integrated nursing team approach. Health Visitor 69: 280–283.

Evaluates the structures, processes, outputs and outcomes of self-managed integrated nursing teams in Essex, which are deemed to have been successful. Key words: staff mix.

Bosma, T. and Higgins, J. (2002) Primary Care Trusts: No can do. Health Service Journal 112(5793): 26–27.

Examines important management issues facing PCTs, including workforce planning. Concentrates on the supply side and educational issues, and especially workforce confederations. Key words: recruitment and retention.

Bowden, H.I. (1987) Manpower planning and health visiting survey. Health Visitor 60: 403–406.

Surveys community managers for their preferred and actual methods for estimating their establishments. Four approaches are described including their strengths and weaknesses. Although the data and results are outmoded the principles apply. Key word: establishments.

Bowling, A. (1985) Management: which tasks can a community nurse take over? Nursing Times 81(43): 46–47.
Bowling, A. (1987) Practice nurses: the future role. Nursing Times 83(17): 31–33.

Explore the early days of nurse practitioners and later after Cumberlege. Look at the development, medicolegal and cost-effectiveness issues. Employment conditions, role and likely future are examined in detail. Data are provided. Organizationally dated but the principles still apply. Key words: staff mix.

Bowns, I.R., Crofts, D.J., Williams, T. et al. (1998) Hitting the Target: A descriptive study of health visitor resource allocation. Sheffield University: SHARR.
Bowns, I.R., Crofts, D.J., Williams, T. et al. (2000) Levels of satisfaction of low risk mothers with their current Health Visitor services. Journal of Advanced Nursing 31: 805–11.

Examine mothers' satisfaction with health visitor services as apart of a broader study of health visitor activity. High levels of satisfaction were found but also scope for improving the level and type of health visitor services. Key words: quality, activity.

Bryar, R. (1994) An examination for the need for new nursing roles in primary healthcare, Journal of Interprofessional Care 8: 73–84.
Bryar, R. (1997) Teamcare valleys – a multifaceted approach to teambuilding in primary health care. In: Pearson, J. and Spencer, J. (eds), Promoting Teamwork in Primary Care. A research based approach. London: Arnold.

Examine current and primary and community practitioner roles and match them to what is needed. Nurse practitioners and public health nursing emerge as the front-runners. Key words: staff mix.

Buchan, J. (1998) Nurse till you drop. Nursing Standard 13(15): 1–5.

Looks at the greying nursing workforce and notes that primary and community care are in a particularly precarious state because these workforces are intrinsically older. Provides a checklist for age-proofing the nursing workforce. Key words: recruitment and retention.

Buchan, J. (1999) The greying of the United Kingdom nursing workforce: implications for employment policy and practice. Journal of Advanced Nursing 30: 818–826.

Detailed and insightful exploration of the ageing nursing workforce. The specific problems for primary and community care managers are highlighted. Explains how continuing professional education tailored for older nurses could help recruitment and retention. Key words: recruitment and retention, education.

Buchan, J. and Edwards, N. (2000) Nursing numbers in Britain: the argument for workforce planning. British Medical Journal 320: 1067–1070.

Explores mostly supply-side workforce planning although demand side gets a fair hearing. Concludes that recruitment and retention on its own is not enough and that workload, workforce size and mix, and integrated workforce planning are imperative. Key words: recruitment and retention, time out.

Buckingham, M. and Wilson, G. (1997) Skill-mix. Use of skill-mix to improve a health visiting service. Health Visiting 70: 267–269.

Explores many structures, processes and some outcomes of an extension of nursery nurses' and Registered Sick Children's Nurses' role towards the work that is normally the health visitor's domain. The new worker's qualifications and experience, supported by appropriate in-service education and supervision, were factors in the project's success. The lack of protocols and guidelines, on the other hand, were a barrier. Key words: staff mix.

Buckle, G. and Gallen, D. (2003) General practice: all in a day's work. Health Service Journal 113(5844): 28–29.

Describes the nature, value and implications of a multidisciplinary first-contact team. The service was judged efficient and effective but the number of self-referrals by patients with self-limiting conditions is worrying. Key words: first contact.

Bull, J. (1998) Integrated nursing: a review of the literature. British Journal of Community Nursing 3: 124–129.

One of the few systematic reviews of integrated community teams. Covers most of their structures, processes and outcomes (skimpy). Key words: staff mix.

Burrell-Davies, L. and Williams, W. (1984) Health visitor manpower survey. Health Visitor 57(1): 9–14.

Profiles the 1980 UK health visitor workforce. Although many health regions did not reply, sufficient did (n = 5) to make the sample representative. Ratios, age, sex, recruitment source and leaver destination are covered in detail. Ample data are provided as well as a pen picture of the 1980s' health visitor workforce. Key word: establishments.

Carlisle, D. (2003) Long division. Health Service Journal 113(5846)(suppl): 4–6.

Summarizes the government's health inequalities policy and strategy. Important data and their sources for health needs analysis are cited. Key words: dependency and acuity.

Cartlidge, A., Bond, J. and Gregson, B. (1987a) Inter professional collaboration. Journal of the Society of Administrators of Family Practice 14: 327–331.

Cartlidge, A., Bond, J. and Gregson, B. (1987b) Inter professional collaboration in primary health care. Nursing Times Occasional Papers 83(6): 45–48.

Discuss the reasons, despite Cumberlege, for the low levels of team work in primary health-care teams. A lack of communication and consultation, which varied between professionals, was the main problem. Organizationally dated but the principles remain. Key words: activity, staff mix.

Chalmers, K. and Kristajanson, L. (1989) The theoretical basis for working at the community level. A comparison of three models. Journal of Advanced Nursing 14: 569–574.

Examines the nature and value of three community care models: (1) public health; (2) community participation; and (3) community change. Key words: activity, public health.

Clark, J. (1984) Mothers' perceptions of health visiting. Health Visiting 57: 265–268.

Longitudinal, qualitative study of health visitor role from the mothers' standpoint. Although the health visitor role was not clear to mothers health visitors' personal attributes were important. Key words: activity, efficiency and effectiveness.

Clews, G. (2003) News focus: weight of expectation. Health Service Journal 113(5842): 10–11.

Delves into the structures and processes behind 24- and 48-hour primary care access targets. Key words: continuing care, first contact.

Clinical Benchmarking Company (1997) Health Visiting Feedback Report. London: CBC.

Historically valuable analysis of health-visiting structures, processes and outcomes. Key words: public health.

Cochrane, D., Conroy, M., Crilly, T. and Rogers, J. (2002) The Future Health Care Workforce. Richmond: Chamberlain Dunn Associates.

Last in the series (two earlier reports) that examines elderly care services, focusing on workforce planning and development. Sticks with the main Future Healthcare Workforce (FHCW) argument – multiskilling and generic working. Key words: staff mix.

Coffey, W. (undated) West Lindsey Dependency Tool. A tool to demonstrate the dependency of patients on the district nursing team. Gainsborough: Lincolnshire District Healthcare NHS Trust.

How-to-do-it manual for measuring community patient dependency. Eleven variables are assessed that place patients in one of three dependency categories ranging from low to high. Vignettes are used to apply the techniques. Key word: dependency.

Cole, A. (2003a) Retirement: into extra time. Health Service Journal 113(5842): 26–28.

Recruitment and retention data that focus on retirement. Recommendations for improving recruitment and retention are soundly based on the data. Key words: recruitment and retention.

Cole, A. (2003b) Violence against staff: government health warning. Health Service Journal 113(5871): 24–25.

Summarizes the National Audit Office report on violent incidents in NHS workplaces. Preventing, handling and reporting violence are considered at length. Community staff are considered a special case. Key words: recruitment and retention.

Colliety, P. (1988a) An evaluation of health visiting process. Part 1. Senior Nurse 8(12): 13–16.
Colliety, P. (1988b) An evaluation of health visiting process. Part 2. Senior Nurse 9(1): 13–16.

Mainly an evaluation of the nursing process applied to health visiting: before and after studies that examine the effects of the health-visiting process on perceptions, activity and satisfaction. Although dated, health-visiting activity data are given that would be useful to someone contemplating an activity analysis. Key words: activity, efficiency and effectiveness.

Collins, K., Jones, M.L., McDonnell, A. et al. (2000) Do new roles contribute to job satisfaction and retention of staff in nursing and professions allied to medicine? Journal of Nursing Management 8: 3–13.

Detailed exploration of job satisfaction and dissatisfaction, which are compared with the broader theoretical and practical public service literature. Key words: recruitment and retention.

Conrane Consulting, NAHAT, Manchester University, et al. (1996) The Future Healthcare Workforce, Manchester: Manchester University.
Conrane Consulting, HSMU and Bournemouth University (1999) The Future Healthcare Workforce: Second Report, University of Bournemouth.

Extend and develop the multiskilling and multiprofessional education debate from the original patient-focused care projects. The shape and size of the NHS workforce needed to meet future health-care needs are discussed in detail. Ample data and examples are provided. Although focused on secondary care, primary and community care are not immune. The second report includes a good section on primary health-care teams. Key word: multiskilling.

Constantinides, P. and Gorden, P. (1990) A model of service. Health Service Journal 100(5222): 1518–1519

Suggests three primary and community care models for London in which nurses feature to varying extents. Pre PCG and PCT. Key words: activity, staff mix.

Cooper, A. (1997) Making skill-mix work. Practice Nurse 13: 521–522.

Describes the planning for and implementation of clinical assistants in primary care. Job descriptions that explain how these assistants work with general and nurse practitioners are included. Education and training are briefly discussed. Key words: staff mix, education and training.

Cotton, L., Brazier, J., Hall, D.M.B. et al. (2000) School nursing: costs and potential benefits. Journal of Advanced Nursing 31: 1063–1071.

Economics-based analysis of school nursing services. Deprivation and children's needs turn out to be a major influence on the establishment and the school nurses' activities. Key words: dependency and acuity.

Coupland, R. (1986) Effective health visiting for elderly people,. Health Visitor 59: 299–300.

Describes the health visitor role caring for elderly patients recently discharged from A&E. Maintaining the elderly person's dependency in the community and raising their quality of life through assessment, intervention and liaison were key tasks. Key words: activity, efficiency and effectiveness.

Cowley, S. (1993) Skill-mix: value for whom? Health Visitor 66: 166–168.

Looks at two broad approaches to primary health-care team workforce planning: the top-down, mechanistic and non-holistic grade-mix approach that leads to grade-mix dilution and cost cutting. Alternatively, the bottom-up, professionally based, intuitive staff-mix approach that can be strengthened using community health needs assessment, which generates a more flexible and potentially cost-effective workforce. Key words: staff mix, dependency and acuity.

Cowley, S. (1995) In health visiting, the routine visit is one that has passed. Journal of Advanced Nursing 22: 276–284.

Revisits the health visitor role empirically and arrives at a set of labels that describe health visitors' therapeutic interventions which are not adequately captured by descriptions of routine surveillance work. Key word: activity.

Cox, A.D., Pound, A., Mills, M. et al. (1991) Evaluation of a home visiting and befriending scheme for young mothers: Newpin. Journal of the Royal Society of Medicine 84: 217–220.

Early in the phase evaluation of young mothers and children with past or current adversity. Results show that befriending schemes by volunteer home workers have a positive influence on these families. Key words: staff mix.

Craig, D. (2003) Chronic Conditions Populations, Management. Northern California: Kaiser Permanente.

Sets out a useful three-group dependency system (from self-help to intensive case management) and associated establishment/staff mix. Staffing is multidisciplinary and generic. Key words: dependency, establishments and staff mix.

Craig, P. and Smith, L. (1998) Health visiting and public health: back to our roots or a new branch. Health and Social Care in the Community 6: 172–180.

Systematic review of the health-visiting role from a historical and contemporary policy perspective. Explores public health roles for health visitors, their strengths and weaknesses. Key words: staff activity.

Craigmile, W.M.N., Fordyce, I. and Mooney, G.H. (1978) Domiciliary care of the elderly. Nursing Times, Occasional Paper 74: 13–15.

Historically valuable data about the structures, processes and outcomes of community care. Key words: continuing care.

Crawford, C.G., Johnson, S.E., Morris, S. et al. (1990) Trent Region District Occupational Therapists Group. Report of the Manpower Planning Project, Sheffield: Trent Regional Health Authority.

Scene-setting document about the issues facing allied health professional workforce planning and development. Key word: establishments.

Crofts, D.J., Bowns, I.R., Williams, T.S. et al. (2000) Hitting the target: the equitable distribution of health visitors across caseloads. Journal of Public Health Medicine 22: 295–301.

Detailed analysis of health visitors' workload predictors, which reveals both expected and unexpected findings regarding caseloads, staffing ratios, mode of working. These vary greatly between areas and the inverse law seems to apply. The time and resources allocated to the care of the child and his or her mother are not always related to need. Key words: dependency, acuity, establishments.

Dalton, E.R., Draper, P.A. and Anderson, J.A. (1972) Changing trends in the staffing levels of community nurses. Community Medicine 128: 97–101.

Examines the theoretical underpinnings and the practical value of nurses per head of population. Even 30 years ago there were illogical discrepancies between districts. Argues that staffing ratios need weighting for accuracy. Outmoded but the principles apply. Key word: establishments.

Daubert, E.A. (1979) Patient classification system and outcome criteria. Nursing Outlook 27: 450–454.

Explores the development of a detailed community–patient dependency classification system. The instrument is based on aims and objectives that should be met by the patient and his or her family carers. Consequently this is useful for evaluating service efficiency and effectiveness as well as establishment setting. Key words: dependency, efficiency and effectiveness.

Davies, J. (2000a) Human resources: finders, keepers. Health Service Journal 110(5733): 24–29.

Précis of the 1999–2000 Department of Health recruitment and retention report and personnel performance reports. Considerable, summarized data are provided, only some of which, however, address primary health specifically. Nevertheless, valuable benchmarks are included. Likely to be superseded by 2001–2 data. Keywords: recruitment and retention.

Davies, J. (2000b) Workforce planning: the devil is in the detail. Health Service Journal 110(5707): 18–21.

Summarizes *A Health Service of All the Talents* and related documents such as the Future Healthcare Workforce. Explains the implications for the NHS workforce and workforce planning. Key words: staff mix.

Deal, L.W. (1994) The effectiveness of community health nursing interventions: a literature review. Public Health Nursing 11: 315–323.

Review of North American community nursing literature. Concentrates on efficiency and effectiveness of mother and toddler care. Explores the rising demand for services and their costs, and the importance of justifying community nursing services based on, for example, health needs and deprivation indicators. Decries the weak design of some studies. Key words: activity, quality, costs.

Denny, E. (1989) The future of health visiting. Health Visitor 62: 250–251.

Reflects on the nature and value of health visiting. Recommends that health visitors review their roles but not get swept along by broader, untested health service changes. Key word: activity.

Department for Education and Skills (2001) National Healthy School Standard. Getting started – a guide for schools (www.wiredforhealth.gov.uk).

Useful information for community child nurses developing school child health programmes. Includes pointers to useful, related sites. Key word: activity.

Department of Health (1993a) Nursing in Primary Care. New world, new opportunities. London: HMSO.

Contemporary and detailed examination about how primary health-care nursing should develop in the light of national health policy. A detailed list of keys to progress offers guidance to practitioners, many of which are relevant today. Key word: activity.

Department of Health (1993b) The Named Nurse, Midwife and Health Visitor. London: HMSO.

Explores the implications of the named primary health-care practitioner. Sections tackle individual practitioner groups such as district and school nursing. Key word: activity.

Department of Health (1993c) The Health of the Nation. Targeting practice. The contribution of nurses, midwives and health visitors. London: DoH.

Discusses *Health of the Nation* targets in a nursing context. Summarizes a number of primary and secondary nursing care projects that address specific targets. Examples from best practice are underlined, which other trusts are encouraged to adopt. Key word: activity.

Department of Health (1993d) The Heathrow Debate. The challenge for nursing and midwifery in the 21st century. London: DoH.

Comprehensive and detailed (24 pages) overview of nursing practice, education and management for the future. Occasionally, specifically concentrates on primary and community care. Organizationally dated. Key word: activity.

Department of Health (1998) Working Together: Securing a quality workforce for the NHS. London: DoH.

Concentrates on broader NHS workforce planning strategies that were introduced in the new NHS White Paper. Sets out workforce planning targets and explores good human resources practice to achieve them. Primary care trusts are the foci. Key word: establishments.

Department of Health (1999a) Making a Difference – Strengthening the nursing, midwifery and health visiting contribution to health and health care. London: DoH.

Discusses nurses and health visitors' roles in the NHS modernization programme, and the challenges they face. Sets out a strategic direction for these practitioners so that they strengthen primary, community and secondary health care services. Key word: activity.

Department of Health (1999b) Recruitment, Retention and Vacancies Survey. London: DoH.

Detailed survey of trusts' recruitment, retention and turnover data analysed mainly by area and by professional group. There are remarkable variations among and between the data. Key words: recruitment and retention.

Department of Health (1999c) Saving Lives: Our healthier nation. London: DoH (www.doh.gov.uk/ohn/popver.htm).

Extends the public health initiative begun in the early 1990s. Concentrates on four health issues: (1) cancer; (2) heart disease and stroke; (3) accidents; and (4) suicide. Explains actions that members of the public can take and how professionals can improve access to health promotion. Has implications for staff mix and health needs assessment. Key words: activity, staff mix, dependency.

Department of Health (2000a) A Health Service of All the Talents. London: DoH.

Examines many demand and supply workforce planning issues. Draws on the Future Healthcare Workforce report (see Conrane Consulting et al. 1996). Examines multi-skilling and multiprofessional education to provide a workforce capable of meeting future health-care demands. Concentrates on the medical workforce but nursing is not ignored. Brutally frank about the inadequacies of the current healthcare workforce-planning framework. Key word: multiskilling.

Department of Health (2000b) Health Select Committee. Future Staffing Requirements. London: DoH.

Summarizes the main issues for reshaping the NHS workforce. Key word: multiskilling.

Department of Health (2001a) Investing and Reform for NHS Staff – Taking forward the plan. London: DoH.

Adds flesh to the strategy set out in *A Health Service of All the Talents*. Five sections logically and clearly set out the issues and actions needed by trusts and related agencies to improve workforce planning and workforce development: (1) increasing staff numbers; (2) recruitment and retention; (3) changing the way staff work; (4) modernizing workforce planning; and (5) investing in staff. Sections are dedicated to primary care. Key words: establishments, recruitment and retention, staff mix.

Department of Health (2001b) Making a Difference in Primary Care: The challenges for nurses, midwifes and health visitors. Case studies from NHS regional conferences. London: DoH (www.doh.gov.uk/nurstrat/primarycare.htm).

Follow on from Department of Health (1999a). Showcases innovative working practices from a wide range of primary and community care services. Key word: activity.

Department of Health (2002a) National Statistics. London: DoH (www.doh.gov.uk).

Comprehensive morbidity, mortality, socioeconomic and demographic tables. Key words: health needs analysis.

Department of Health (2002b) Primary Care Workforce Planning Framework (www.doh.gov.uk/pricare/pcwf.htm).

Comprehensive and highly usable report that sets out the ingredients and methods of primary and community care workforce planning/development in two main sections: (1) introduction, background and context, and (2) planning and developing a workforce to meet the needs of the future. Plenty of signposts are included that direct the reader to helpful websites and agencies. Key words: activity, education and training, quality and costs, recruitment and retention, staff mix.

Department of Health (2002c) Liberating the Talents. London: DoH (www.doh.gov.uk/cnoliberatingtalents).

Consolidates recent Department of Health policies to advise and guide primary and community care workforce planners. The new framework for primary and community nursing describes three new primary nursing functions: (1) first contact: assessment, diagnosis, treatment and referral; (2) continuing care: disease management and rehabilitation; and (3) public health: health protection and promotion. Good practice examples are provided. Key words: activity, staff mix.

Department of Health (2002d) Essence of Care. London: DoH (ww.doh.gov.uk/essenceofcare).

Provides best practice benchmarks on aspects that are central to the quality of patient care. Key word: quality.

Department of Health (2002e) NSF Diabetes: Delivery strategy. London: DoH (www.doh.gov.uk/nsf/diabetes/delivery/ch6/workforce-planning.htm).
Department of Health (2002f) Workforce Matters. A guide to role redesign in diabetes. London: DoH.

Chapter 6 looks at the workforce issues regarding the NSF for Diabetes. Discussion is more strategic than operational and other websites/documents are signposted. Key words: skill mix and grade mix.

Department of Health (2002g) Executive Summary: NSF for older people. London: DoH (doh.gov.uk/nsf/olderpeople.htm).

One section reminds the reader about the NSF workforce-planning framework before discussing elderly care workforce planning and development issues. Key words: continuing care.

Department of Health (2003) Liberating the Public Health Talents of Community Practitioners and Health Visitors. London: DoH.

Updates *Liberating the Talents* and concentrates on community practitioners. Includes case studies and examples of good practice. Key words: staff activity.

Department of Health (2004) Agenda for Change: What will it mean for you? A guide for staff. London: DoH.

Detailed update on the new pay and reward scheme for NHS staff. Key word: personnel.

Dewis, S. (2001) Nottingham Community Health District Caseload Review Project. Hucknall: Broxtowe and Hucknall PCT.

A detailed analysis of one health authority's community nursing workforce. Dependency, acuity and activity are explored in detail. Considerable data are provided for benchmarking results. Key words: dependency, acuity and activity.

Dobby, J. (1986) The Development and Testing of a Method for Measuring the Need for, and the Value of Routine Health Visiting Within a District Health Authority. London: Health Promotion Research Unit.

Dobby, J. and Barnes, A. (1987a) Measuring the need for and the value of routine health visiting – 1. Health Visitor 60(2): 81–82.

Dobby, J. and Barnes, A. (1987b) Measuring the need for and the value of routine health visiting – 2. Health Visitor 60(3): 114–115.

Part 1 examines the actual and potential health visitor role. It decries the paucity of information for assessing the need for and evaluating the effectiveness of health visiting. Suggests one approach for correcting this deficiency. Part 2 extends this approach from those aged 0–5 to older patients. Key words: dependency, quality.

Drennan, V. (1990a) Gathering information from the field. Nursing Times 86(39): 46–48.

Drennan, V. (1990b) Striving for fairer workloads. Nursing Times 86(40): 48–49.

Theoretical and practical examination of the variables contributing to district nurse patient dependency and acuity. Describe how instruments were generated, and how data were collected and used to profile, benchmark and change practice. Few data are provided, however. Organizationally outdated but the principles are strong. Key words: activity, dependency, acuity.

Durrand, I. (1989) Nurse/patient dependency in community nursing. Nursing Times, Occasional Paper 85(5): 55–57.

Describes the literature basis, construction, piloting and application of community patient dependency and acuity measures. More theoretical than practical. Dated but the principles survive. Key words: literature review, dependency, acuity.

Earl-Slater, A. (1995) Management review: Coventry's fast response service cuts hospital stays. British Journal of Health Care Management 1: 596–599.

Describes one health authority's forerunner to the modern-day Intensive Home Support Scheme, which assesses patients' needs, provides suitable services through a network of health and social services with the aim of maintaining patients in the community. Key words: activity, staff mix.

Ebeid, A. (2000) Primary care: staff-mix development in health visiting: meeting the agenda, Community Practitioner 73: 687–689.

Describes how staff mix was reviewed and changed in one London health authority. Honestly reports the upsides and downsides of changing grade and staff mix. Organizationally dated but the principles survive. Key words: staff mix.

Editorial (1997) Delegation and referral in primary health care teams. Nursing Standard 11(49): 32–33.

Summarizes the Jenkins-Clarke et al. (1997) report. Highlights the delegation, teamwork and patient satisfaction issues. Key words: staff mix.

Edwardson, S.R. and Nardone, P. (1990) The dependency at discharge instrument as a measure of resource use in home care. Public Health Nursing 7: 138–144.

Psychometrically robust study of a community patient dependency measure. Goes on to relate dependency to acuity and health-care resource groups. Warns of the dangers of delivering services irrationally. Key words: dependency, acuity, costs.

Eli Lilly National Clinical Audit Centre (1992) A Method of Surveying Patient Satisfaction. Instructions for MAAGS. Leicester University: Department of General Practice.

How-to-do-it pack using general practice patient satisfaction surveys (consultation satisfaction and surgery satisfaction questionnaires). Includes benchmarks along Maxwellian lines that help practice staff to compare themselves. Key word: quality.

Elkan, R., Kendrick, D., Hewitt, M. et al. (2000a) The effectiveness of domiciliary health visiting: a systematic review of international studies and a selective review of the British literature. Health Technology Assessment 4: 340.

Elkan, R., Robinson, J.J.A. and Blair, M. (2000b) Evidence-based practice and health visiting: the need for theoretical underpinnings for evaluation. Journal of Advanced Nursing 31: 1316–1323.

Elkan, R., Robinson, J.J.A., Blair, M. et al. (2000c) The effectiveness of health services: the case of health visiting. Health and Social Care in the Community 8: 70–78.

Extensive meta-analysis and systematic literature reviews. Comprehensive exploration of health visiting and health-care assistant roles, health needs assessment, practice models, cost-effectiveness and quality of care. Raise many new questions about the health-visiting workforce as well as underlining their worth. Look at theoretical models that can be used to explain health-visiting structures, processes and outcomes. Relate these to evidence-based practice, measurement and application. Key words: efficiency and effectiveness, literature review, quality, activity.

Elliott, L., Crombie, I.K., Irvine, L. et al. (2004) Methodological issues in nursing research. The effectiveness of public health nursing: the problem and solution in carrying out a review of systematic reviews. Journal of Advanced Nursing 45: 117–125.

The highs and lows of systematically studying public health nursing literature are explored – mostly about how to do this, although operational and strategic issues emerge for workforce planners and developers. Key words: staff activity.

Evers, H., Badger, F., Cameron, E. et al. (1991a) Taking extra care. Health Service Journal 101(5259): 27.

Evers, H., Badger, F., Cameron, E. et al. (1991b) Who should do the housework? Health Service Journal 101(5260): 22–23.

Thoughtful examination of the dividing line between community nurses and local authority carers' roles. Clarify which roles belong to whom and propose a category of work called 'extra care', which community nurses carry out on behalf of local authority carers. Key words: activity, staff mix.

Fatchett, A. and Gleeson, C. (2002) Child health. School nursing – proving the value. Primary Health Care 12(6): 24–25.

Examines the nature and value of school nurses' roles using focus groups. Recommends that school nurses' roles are strengthened. Key word: activity.

Fitton, J.M. (1984a) Health visiting the elderly: nurse managers' views 1. Nursing Times, Occasional Paper 80, 16(10): 59–61.
Fitton, J.M. (1984b) Health visiting the elderly: nurse managers' views 2. Nursing Times, Occasional Paper 80, 17(11): 67–69.

Argue from an empirical basis about the health visitor's role especially for the care of elderly people. Many saw barriers to maintaining comprehensive services that spanned the full age range. Organizationally dated but the principles apply. Key word: activity.

Frame, G. and O'Donnell, P. (1996) Community nursing: weight lifters. Health Service Journal 106(5224): 30–31.

Describes and tests a specimen community patient dependency scoring system. Data are provided. Key words: dependency and acuity.

Gerrish, K., Ross, B. and Thompson, V. (1998) Primary healthcare: reviewing responsibilities. Journal of Clinical Nursing 12(10): 1–9.

Discusses maximizing district nurses' contribution. Reviews the responsibilities of different grades of community nurse. Key words: activity, staff mix.

Gibbing, S. (1995) Dependency, skill-mix and grade-mix and their effects on health visiting practice. Journal of Clinical Nursing 4: 43–47.

Compares and contrasts dependency in primary and secondary settings. Provides insights into the interrelationship of dependency, establishments, and skill/grade mix. No methods or staffing data are provided. Key words: grade/staff mix.

Gleeson, C. (2003) Clinical: young people. Improving teenagers' access to health services. Practice Nursing 14: 263–266.
Gleeson, C., Robinson, M. and Neal, R. (2002) A review of teenagers' perceived needs and access to primary health care: implications for health services. Primary Health Care Research 3: 184–193.

Look at the relationship between practice nurses and teenage patients. Raise the potential problems and offer solutions. Key word: activity.

Goldacre, M. (1998) Planning the United Kingdom's medical workforce. British Medical Journal 316: 1846–1847.

Examines medical workforce supply and demand issues. Key words: establishments, recruitment and retention.

Goldstone, L. and Worrall, J. (1980) The problem of variations in work patterns of district nurses. Nursing Times, Occasional Paper 76(11): 45–51.

Explains some remarkable variations in community nursing activity using activity analysis. Recommends that community patient dependency and workload measurement become commonplace. Key words: dependency–acuity and activity.

Goldstone, L.A., Wing, S., Barker, L. and Hughes, A. (2000) But who will make the visits? A patient-related information system for management in district nursing. Health Informatics Journal 6: 39–44.

Applies an acuity–quality workforce planning method to the community. Suggests how the system can be used to indicate workload and evaluate the size and mix of district nursing teams. Key words: dependency–acuity, quality, establishments.

Goodman, C. (1996) District nursing and the NHS reforms: a case for clarification. Journal of Nursing Management 4(40): 1–9.

Systematic review of the district nursing commissioning literature. Explores the reasons why district nurses do not fully participate in the purchasing and commissioning. Key words: activity, literature review.

Goodwin, S. (1988) Whither Health Visiting? London: Health Visitors' Association

Comprehensive examination of health visiting theory and practice. Outmoded but many principles still apply. Key word: activity.

Goodwin, S. (1994) Purchasing effective healthcare for parents and young children. Health Visitor 67: 127–129.

Comprehensive look at evidence-based purchasing of primary and community services. Community staffing structures, processes and outcomes are explored. Organizationally dated but the principles apply today. Key words: health needs assessment.

Harrogate Centre for Excellence in Health and Social Care (2003) Conference Pack: Developing the role of first contact nursing. improving access, assessment and choice. Meeting the targets. Harrogate: HCEHSC (www.hmc.co.uk).

Early exploration of First Contact nursing issues. Speakers' notes are available. Key words: staff activity, staff mix.

Healy, P. (2002a) Traditional role will go in overhaul of primary care. Nursing Standard 17(7): 5.
Healy, P. (2002b) Primary care will make nurses first contact. Nursing Standard 17(10): 5.

Briefly describe the background, rationale, history, nature and purpose of *Liberating the Talents*. Key words: staff mix, staff activity.

Heath, I. (1994) Skill mix in primary care. British Medical Journal 308: 993–994.

Reflects on actual primary and community care staff mix and the recommendations in the value for money (VFM) report (NHS Management Executive 1992). Dated but the principles apply. Key words: staff mix.


Hesketh, J. (2002) The district nursing workforce: so where do we go from here? British Journal of Nursing 11: 526.

Briefly explores primary and community workforce planning and development in the light of health and changing health and social care. Key word: establishments.


Hill, L. and Rutter, L. (2001) Primary care trusts: cut to the quick. Health Service Journal 111(5775): 24–25.

Describes a multifaceted approach to improving patient access to primary (and secondary) care. These new approaches extend nursing roles. Key words: first contact, continuing care.


Hirst, M., Lunt, N. and Atkin, K. (1998) Were practice nurses distributed equitably across England and Wales, 1988–1995? Journal of Health Services Research and Policy 3: 31–38.

Examines the reasons behind the growth of practice nursing, its implications and irrational basis for the growth, e.g. there is not always a relationship between workforce growth and locality's need. Key word: staff mix.


Hodder, P. (1995) Towards an integrated primary health care team. Value for Money Update 1: 6–7.

Describes a pilot that shows the nature and value of the integrated primary health-care team. Explains the implications for roll out. Organizationally dated but the principles apply. Key words: integrated teams.


Holland, K. (1998) Integrated nursing team evaluation, unpublished dissertation, Leeds University, Nuffield Institute for Health.

Detailed, empirical evaluation of the structures, processes and outcomes of integrated, self-managed community teams. Key words: grade/staff mix.


Howkins, E. and Thornton, C. (2003) Editorial: liberating the talents: whose talents and for what purpose? Journal of Nursing Management 11: 219–220.

An early critique of *Liberating the Talents*, raising managerial and political questions about this new policy. Lack of space probably prevented the authors from exploring the three main *Liberating the Talents* components: first contact, continuing care and public health. Key word: activity.

Hudson, M. and Hawthorn, P. (1989) Clinical: stroke patients at home: who cares? Nursing Times 85(22): 48–50

Analyses the type and pattern of care of stroke patients by district nurses. Inappropriate working is discussed at length. Dated findings but the principles apply. Key words: staff activity.

Hurst, K. (2003) Estimating the Size and Mix of Nursing Teams. Leeds: Nuffield Institute and Department of Health.

Executive summary of a large report that describes the nature and value of five main inpatient workforce planning methods. The professional judgement method has the most relevance to the primary and community workforce. Key word: establishments.

Hurst, K., Ford, J. and Gleeson, C. (2002) Evaluating self-managed integrated community teams. Journal of Management in Medicine 16: 463–483.

Detailed evaluation of self-managed integrated teams (SMITs). Includes a systematic review of the literature, results of surveys of practitioners' perceptions of SMIT structures, processes and outcomes. Survey data are compared with observation, interview and focus group data from the same context. Workforce planning and development are well covered. Although many positive findings emerge, barriers to effective SMITs still give managers and practitioners problems. Workforce planning and development are well covered. Key words: integrated teams, establishments, efficiency and effectiveness, education and training.

Hyatt, E. (2003) What blocks health visitors from taking on a leadership role? Journal of Nursing Management 11: 229–233.

Examines health visitors' power to influence and lead primary and community service change. Some peripheral aspects such as the supply and demand for primary care trusts are also covered. Key words: establishments, activity, efficiency and effectiveness.

Hyde, V. (ed.) (2001) Community Nursing and Health Care Innovations and Insights. London: Arnold.

State-of-the-art review of issues impinging on community nursing. Covers health care needs, workforce issues, education and legal developments. Key words: establishments, staff mix, education and training.

Illsley, V.A. and Goldstone, L.A. (1986) Management: measuring quality in district nursing. Nursing Times 82(27): 38–40.
Illsley, V.A. and Goldstone, L.A. (1987) District Nursing Monitor: An index of the quality of nursing care for patients of the district nursing service. Newcastle-upon-Tyne: Newcastle-upon-Tyne Polytechnic Publications.
Illsley, V. and Goldstone, L.A. (1992) District Nursing Monitor 2. Newcastle: Unique Business Service Press.

Easily the most comprehensive community nursing quality assessment measure. The outmoded elements have been revised in the second edition. The *Nursing Times* article describes the authors' preparatory work and the implications for document-based quality assurance systems for community care. Key words: efficiency and effectiveness.

Jeffreys, L., Clark, A.L. and Kaperski, M. (1995) Practice nurses' workload and consultation patterns. British Journal of General Practice 45: 415–418.

Detailed analysis of practice nurse activity and judgements about their efficiency and effectiveness. Key words: activity, efficiency and effectiveness

Jenkins-Clarke, S. (1997) Delegation and referral in primary health care teams. Nursing Standard 11(49): 32–33.
Jenkins-Clarke, S. and Carr-Hill, R. (1996) Discussion Paper 144: Measuring skill-mix in primary care: dilemmas of delegation and diversification. York University: Centre for Health Economics.
Jenkins-Clarke, S. and Carr-Hill, R. (2001) Changes, challenges and choices for the primary healthcare workforce: looking to the future. Journal of Advanced Nursing 34: 842–849.
Jenkins-Clarke, S., Carr-Hill, R., Dixon, P. and Pringle, M. (2001a) Skill Mix in Primary Care. Executive Summary. York University: Centre for Health Economics.
Jenkins-Clarke, S., Carr-Hill, R. and Dixon, P. (2001b) Teams and seams: skill-mix in primary care. Journal of Advanced Nursing 28: 1120–1126.

Series of papers that look at the upsides and downsides of delegation in primary care. Methods are discussed at length. Results consider policy issues and the ideal primary health-care team staff mix. Inappropriate working is also discussed along with staff attitudes and perceptions. Patient satisfaction with consultations is included. Key words: staff mix, efficiency and effectiveness, activity.

Kelsey, A. (1995) Outcome measures: problem and opportunities for public health nurses. Journal of Nursing Management 3: 183–187.

Clear and focused discussion about specifying and measuring public health nursing outcomes. Recommends two measuring approaches, including their strengths and weaknesses. Key words: efficiency and effectiveness.

Kelsey, A. and Robinson, M. (1999) 'But they don't see the whole child . . .' health visitors may not welcome systematic review of child health surveillance. British Journal of General Practice 49: 4–5.

Explores the influence systematic reviews may have on health visitor establishments and working practice. Argues that analysis of solitary variables does not adequately describe health visitors' holistic role and the multiskilling capability. Key word: activity.

Kemp, I.W. (1969) Health visiting in Scotland. Health Bulletin 27(2): 21–29.

Historically valuable account of health visiting structures, processes and outcomes. Key words: public health.

Kendall, L. and Lissauer, R. (eds) (2003) The Future Health Worker. London: IPPR.

State-of-the-art review of NHS workforce planning and development. Important policy and practice issues are considered in detail. Wide-ranging evidence is used to support and refute current perceptions of the NHS workforce. Doctor centred, although nursing and therapy are discussed in all health settings. Several recommendations are made to help plan and develop the future health-care workforce. Key words: staff mix.

Kendrick, D., West, J., Wright, S. et al. (1995) Does routine child health surveillance reach children most at risk of accidental injury? Journal of Public Health Medicine 17: 39–45.

Detailed and robust study of child accidents and the variables that predict accidents. Health visitor role is important because the findings show that prioritizing families from high to low need/risk is likely to help health visitors monitor children at risk. Key words: health needs assessment.

Klein, L. and Tomlinson, P. (1987a) Patchwork. Nursing Times 83(26): 39–40.
Klein, L. and Tomlinson, P. (1987b) Sharing the caring. Nursing Times 83(27): 60–61.

Explore health-visiting establishments based on deprivation and other health-care needs data. Organizationally dated but principles remain active. Key words: staff mix

Kneafsey, R., Long, A.F. and Ryan, J. (2003) An exploration of the contribution of the community nurse to rehabilitation. Health and Social Care in the Community 11: 321–328.

Deep qualitative enquiry into community nurses' actual and perceived role in community rehabilitation. Considers missed opportunities, education and training, de-skilling and multidisciplinary team working. Key words: activity, staff mix.

Lancaster and South Cumbria Education and Training Consortium (1998) Clinical Placements for PAMs. Lancaster: LSCETC and NHS Executive North West.

Sets out allied health professional education and training issues. Keywords: education and training

Latimer, J. and Ashburner, L. (1997) Primary care nursing. How can nurses influence its development? NT Researcher 2: 258–267.

Detailed literature review-based examination of primary care nursing developments. Looks at many workforce planning issues including education and training, mutidisciplinary working and cross-training, support, development and service fragmentation. Key words: staff mix.

Lauder, W.A. (1999) A survey of self-neglect in patients living in the community. Journal of Clinical Nursing 8: 95–102.

Examines the psychological and physical differences between self-neglecting patients and a control group. Notes that self-neglecting patients in the community are not necessarily highly dependent. Key word: dependency.

Leach, P. (1997) What price home visiting and family support? Health Visitor 70(2): 72–74.

Anecdotal, personal account of diminishing home visiting services. Key word: activity

Ledger, P. (1987) A review of Health Visitor establishments at a health centre and a GP practice. Health Visitor 60(9): 30–33.
Ledger, P. (1988) Feasibility study for evening, night and weekend health visiting. Health Visitor 61(3): 71–72.

Related articles that look at health-visiting establishments broadly including health-care needs based and workload. Set out studies showing that health visitors out of hours were not wanted by patients nor was it deemed cost-effective. Staffing formulae and data are given. Organizationally dated but the principles survive. Key words: activity, staffing.

Leeds Community and Mental Health Services Teaching NHS Trust (2001) Improving Working Lives Survey. Leeds: LCMHT.

Publishes the results of one trust's efforts at the *Improving Working Lives* staff survey requirement. Job satisfaction and workload are two relevant areas covered. Key words: recruitment and retention.

Lewis, C. (2003a) Clinical management: full team ahead. Health Service Journal 113(5871): 28–29.

Changing workforce approach to re-designing diabetes care. Efficiency and effectiveness have been improved by developing the diabetic nurse specialist, technician and other roles. Roll out to other chronic disease management issues is planned. Key words: activity, staff mix.

Lewis, C. (2003b) Clinical management: measure of success. Health Service Journal 113(5884): 28–29.

A framework in which to think and act when measuring and monitoring public health. Relates well to *Liberating the Talents*. Key word: activity

Lewis, R. and deBene, J. (1994) Substitution: a switch in time. Health Service Journal 104(5408): 30–32.

Considers the community resources needed for transferring hospital to community care. Skill-mix, equipment, education and training are singled out. Organizationally dated but the principles survive. Key words: staff mix.

Lewis, R. and Rosen, R. (2003) The American way. Health Service Journal 113(5874): 30–31.

Generates valuable insights into chronic disease management by comparing North American managed care with UK Personal Medical Service and General Medical Service. Key word: activity.

Lightfoot, J. (1993) Nursing by numbers. Health Service Journal 103(5874): 26–27.

Lightfoot, J., Baldwin, S. and Wright, K. (1992) Nursing by Numbers: Setting staffing levels for district nursing and health visiting services. York University: Social Policy Research Unit.

Look at the methods, data and limitations to measuring community nursing workload by exploring the rationale for setting community establishments using actual and projected geographic, demographic and socioeconomic data. Organizationally dated but principles survive. Key word: establishments.

Lissauer, R. and Kendall, L. (eds) (2002) New Practitioners in the Future Health Service. Exploring roles for practitioners in primary and intermediate care. London: IPPR.

State-of-the-art review of NHS workforce planning and development. Important policy and practice issues are considered in detail. Wide-ranging evidence is used to support and refute current perceptions of the NHS workforce. Doctor centred, although nursing and therapy are discussed in all health settings. Several recommendations are made to help plan and develop the future health-care workforce. Key words: staff mix.

Lochead, E. (1994) Introducing nursery nurses to the school health team. Health Visitor 67(4): 133–134.

One of the few articles that explores school nursing establishments. No data or algorithms are provided. Organizationally dated but the principles survive. Key word: establishments.

Long, A.F., Kneafsey, R., Ryan, L. et al. (2002) The role of the nurse within the multiprofessional rehabilitation team. Journal of Advanced Nursing 37: 70–78.

Provides a framework for acute and community nursing. Underlines nurses' role in rehabilitation and what can be done to strengthen their role. Key word: activity.

Luft, S. (1990) Community: measuring patient dependency nursing. Nursing 4(9): 13–16.

Describes the development and application of a community–patient dependency-rating instrument. Specimen data are provided but psychometric properties are not discussed. Key word: dependency.

McDonald, A., Langford, I. and Boldeno, N. (1997) The future of community nursing in the United Kingdom: district nursing, health visiting and school nursing. Journal of Advanced Nursing 26: 257–265.

Empirically based review of primary and community nursing. Explores actual and desired roles, inappropriate working, staff-mix changes, education and training. Organizationally dated but the principles survive. Key words: staff mix, activity.

McDonald, P. (1996) Can timed appointments for community staff improve care? Nursing Times 92(18): 35–37.

Focuses on the strengths and weaknesses of timed domiciliary community practitioners' visits. Key words: cost, quality, continuing care.

McIntosh, J.B. and Richardson, I.M. (1976) Report 37: Work Study of District Nursing Staff. Edinburgh: Scottish Home and Health Department.

Detailed theoretical and practical study of community patient dependency and acuity. Dated but the principles survive. Key words: dependency and acuity.

McIntosh, J., Moriarty, D., Lugton, J. et al. (2000) Evolutionary change in the use of skills within the district nursing team: a study in two Health Board Areas in Scotland. Journal of Advanced Nursing 32: 783–790.

Ethnographic exploration of district nursing practice from a grade- and staff-mix perspective. Concentrates on inappropriate working, delegation, leadership and supervision. Key words: staff activity, staff mix.

Mackenzie, A. and Ross, F. (1997) Shifting the balance of nursing in primary care. British Journal of Community Health Nursing 2(3): 139–142.

Examines primary nursing care following the introduction of primary care groups and trusts. Broad ranging review including clinical, managerial and educational issues. Organizationally dated but principles survive. Key word: activity.

Maggs, C.J. (1995) The Follow-up Report: District Nursing Direct Patient Care Contact Workload, Cardiff University: Department of Nursing Research.
Maggs, C.J. and Rapport, F.L. (1994) District Nursing Direct Patient Care Contact Workload, Cardiff University: Department of Nursing Research.

Qualitative study of district nurses' perceptions about their work and changing primary care, management and practice. Practitioner views are compared with those of managers and the differences noted. Recommendations are made to improve district nurses' working lives and the quality of patient care. See also Rapport and Maggs (1997). Key word: activity.

Malone, C. and Mackenzie, R. (2000) Community care: in the know. Health Service Journal 110(5721): 28–29.

Considers the implications of a growing elderly population and the lack of experienced nurses in care homes. Notes the nursing problems that arise from care homes and offers solutions to ease the additional workload falling on community nurses. Key words: staff activity.

Martin, C. (1987) Practice nurses: practice makes perfect? Nursing Times 83(17): 28–31.

Dated but comprehensive review of practice nursing around the time of Cumberlege. Highlights unusual differences between practice nurses and other members of the health care team and the implications of practice nurses' closer working relationship with GPs. Key words: staff activity.

Mathie, T. (2002) Overseas recruitment: the Spanish acquisitions. Health Service
    Journal 112(5834): 28–29.
Mathie, T. and McKinley, D. (1999) A GP Recruitment Survey in the North West
    Region. London: DoH

Look at recruitment and retention variables in the north west. The impact on primary
and community nursing emerges. Key words: recruitment and retention.


Meadows, S., Levenson, R. and Baeza, J. (2000) The Last Straw. London: King's Fund.

Detailed empirical examination of nursing recruitment and retention issues. Includes a
comprehensive literature review of: public view of nursing; nursing roles; positive recruitment and retention; negative recruitment and retention; gender; education and training;
organization issues. Key words: recruitment and retention.


Medical Practices Committee (2001) Skill-mix in Primary Care – Implications for
    the future. London: MPC.

Comprehensive, constructively critical review of primary care demand and supply-side
staffing and mix. Delegation, substitution, recruitment and retention are considered at
length. GP focused with only cursory mentions of other primary health-care trust
members. Key words: staff mix, recruitment and retention.


Moody, L. (2003) Primary care: those who can. Health Service Journal 113(5844): 30.

Sets out one primary care trust's response to worsening primary and community care
recruitment and retention. Initiatives include careful workforce, multidisciplinary, first
contact, enhanced NVQs, cadet and GP with special interest schemes. Key words: recruitment and retention.


Moran-Ellis, J., Battle, S. and Salter, B. (1985) A day in the life of a DN. Nursing
    Times Community Outlook 81: 42.

Organizationally dated but useful examination of district nursing activity based on a comprehensive review of care. Concludes that some personal care activities are
inappropriately carried out by highly skilled district nurses. Key words: staff activity.


Naish, J. and Kline, R. (1990) What counts can't always be counted. Health Visitor
    63: 421–422.

Dated but thorough exploration of contracting and its relationship to workforce planning
and service quality. Argues that hard data may not be the answer and that softer data have
an important part to play. Key words: efficiency and effectiveness.


National Primary and Care Trust Organisation or NatPaCT (2002a)
    Demonstrators: Professional Development Regulation (www.natpact.nhs.uk).
NatPaCT (2002b) The Organisational Competency Framework (www.natpact.
    nhs.uk).

Organizational competency assessment tool with nine themes designed to help primary care trust managers. The framework is evolving and incomplete at the last check. However, workforce planning features strongly. Key word: personnel.

NHS Executive (2000a) Improving Working Lives. Programmes for change. Leeds: NHS Executive.

Builds on the workforce planning strategies set out in *Securing a quality workforce for the NHS* (DoH 1998). Key word: establishments.

NHS Executive (2000b) Recruiting and Retaining Nurses, Midwives and Health Visitors in the NHS – A progress report. Leeds: NHS Executive.

Review of progress made on improving recruitment and retention. Most if not all the important recruitment and retention variables are explored. Case studies exemplifying best practice are included, which make community and primary care nursing explicit. Key words: recruitment and retention.

NHS Management Executive (1992) Value for Money Unit Report: Nursing skill-mix in the district nursing service. Leeds: NHS Executive.

Used activity sampling in three community units. Controversially recommended a 50% dilution of community nursing grade mix because too many H and G grade nurses worked inappropriately. Key words: staff mix.

NHS Workforce Taskforce, HR Directorate and Department of Health (2002) HR in the NHS Plan. London: DoH (www.doh.gov.uk).

Sets out human resource best practice in the context of *The NHS Plan*. Concentrates on the supply side; however, multiskilling and staff mix are briefly considered. The four human resource pillars, skills escalator and modernization are considered. Key words: staff mix, recruitment and retention.

Nicholson, P. (1998) Managing workload. Skill mix: a pilot study within a health visiting team. Community Practitioner 71(5): 175–176.

Examines paediatric nurses' contribution to community nursing, particularly health visiting. Key words: staff mix.

Noakes, B. and Johnson, N. (1999) Primary care: don't leave me this way. Health Service Journal 109(5465): 20–21.

Analyses current workforce planning and development issues and their likely implications for primary care trusts. Empirically strong and provides valuable primary care data and guidance not often found in national databases. Key word: methods.

Obeid, A. (1997) The district/practice nurse mix. Nursing Management 3(9): 17–18.

Argues for the integration of practice and district nursing to improve efficiency and effectiveness as well as solving recruitment and retention problems. Underlines the barriers and challenges facing managers wishing to adjust staff mix along these lines. Key words: staff mix.

Ong, B.N. (1991) Researching needs in district nursing. Journal of Advanced Nursing 16: 638–647.

Theoretical exploration of patients' and carers' needs, and professionals' views of services. Although both quantitative and qualitative methods were used, the latter predominate. There was no dissonance between the three groups but patients' and carers' views provide useful insights. Key words: efficiency and effectiveness.

Patterson, J. (2003) Primary care: central reservations. Health Service Journal 113(5838): 30–31.

Examines emerging primary and community workforce planning issues. Key word: activity.

Phillip, L.R., Morrison, E.F. and Chae, Y.M. (1990) The QUALCARE scale: developing an instrument to measure quality of home care, International Journal of Nursing Studies 27(1): 61–75.

Elderly care quality measured using an instrument similar to quality patient care scale. North American derivation, so some of the six elements do not sit comfortably in the UK. Psychometrically robust, comprehensive measure of care in the elderly patient's or carer's home. Key words: efficiency and effectiveness.

Piggott, M. (1988) Making the numbers add up. Nursing Times 84(1): 36–37.

Sets out the principles for determining health-visiting workload using predominantly family socioeconomic factors, although clinical issues are not ignored. Key word: workload.

Plews, C., Billingham, K. and Rowe, A. (2000) Public health nursing: barriers and opportunities. Health and Social Care in the Community 8(2): 1–11.

Qualitative and quantitative study of managers' and practitioners' perceptions of public health nursing. The reasons for the current state of primary care are explained along with solutions for strengthening public health nursing. Key word: activity.

Poulton, B.C. (1996) Use of the consultation satisfaction questionnaire to examine patients' satisfaction with general practitioner and community nurses: reliability, replicability and discriminant validity. British Journal of General Practice 46: 26–31.

Detailed examination of community patient satisfaction questionnaire psychometric issues. Key word: quality.

Poulton, B. (1995) Effective multidisciplinary teamwork in primary care, unpublished PhD thesis, Sheffield University.

Poulton, B. and West, M. (1993) Effective multidisciplinary teamwork in primary care. Journal of Advanced Nursing 18: 918–925.

Poulton, B.C. and West, M.A. (1994) Primary care team effectiveness: developing a constituency approach. Community 2: 77–84.

Largely theoretical discussion of efficient and effective primary health teamwork. Includes a discussion of staff mix and quality of care. Organizationally dated but the principles and models survive. Key words: staff mix.

Poulton, K. (1977) Community Nursing Service at Wansworth and East Merton Teaching District. London: South West Thames Regional Health Authority.

Poulton, K. (1984) A measure of independence. Nursing Times 80(34): 32–35.

Describe an empirically determined dependency and acuity rating system for the elderly in care homes and the patient's home. Key words: dependency and acuity.

Prideaux, R. (1996) A method of skill-mix. Journal of Community Nursing 10(4): 16–18.

Sets the size and mix of community teams using patient dependency and nursing activity. Results show that grade mix was dilute. Changes were successfully made largely as a result of the top-down and bottom-up method. Key words: staff mix.

Proctor, S. and Campbell, J. (1999) A developmental performance framework for primary care. International Journal of Healthcare Quality Assurance 12: 279–286.

Theoretical and empirically based study of primary care quality and performance. Examines quality from users' and professionals' perspective. Key words: efficiency and effectiveness.

Rapport, F. and Maggs, C. (1997) Measuring care: the case of district nursing. Journal of Advanced Nursing 25: 673–680.

Qualitative study of district nurses' perceptions about their work and changing primary care, management and practice. Practitioner views are compared with managers' views and the differences noted. Recommendations are made to improve district nurses' working lives and the quality of patient care. See also Maggs and Rapport (1994) and Maggs (1995). Key word: activity.

Rashid, A., Watts, A., Levenham, C. et al. (1996) Skill in primary care: sharing clinical workload and understanding professional roles. British Journal of General Practice 46: 639–240.

Literature-based reflection of GP team mix that concentrates on nurse practitioner roles. Key words: staff mix.

Reading, R. and Allen, C. (1997) The impact of social inequalities in child health on health visitors' work. Journal of Public Health Medicine 19: 424–430.

Exploration of health-visiting workload and activity based on detailed, empirical socioeconomic data. Concludes that health visitor activity is not always related to families in need. Key word: dependency.

Richards, A., Carley, J., Jenkins-Clarke, S. and Richards, D.A. (2000) Skill mix between nurses and doctors working in primary care delegation or allocation: a review of the literature. International Journal of Nursing Studies 37: 185–197.

Recent and comprehensive systematic review of primary care staff mix in a context of delegation. Examines GP and practice nurse activity and workload, advanced practice, delegation, education and training, teamwork and patient satisfaction. An extensive list of citations is included. Key words: staff mix, activity, education and training and patient satisfaction.

Richardson, G. (1999) Identifying, evaluating and implementing cost-effective skill-mix. Journal of Advanced Nursing 7: 265–270.

Richardson, G. and Maynard, A. (1995) Discussion Paper 3: Fewer Doctors? More Nurses? A Review of the Knowledge Base of Doctor–Nurse Substitution. York University: Centre for Health Economics.

Richardson, G., Maynard, A., Cullum, N. et al. (1998) Skill mix changes: substitution or service development? Health Policy 45: 119–132.

Systematic review of the literature from a labour substitution angle. Look at staff mix from a cost–benefit and other economic perspectives. Questions the cost-effectiveness of skills substitution from doctors to nurses. Discuss some supply-side workforce variables that complicate the staff-mix situation. Key words: staff mix.

Rink, E., Ross, F., Godfrey, E. et al. (1996) The changing use of nursing skills in general practice. British Journal of Community Health Nursing 1: 364–369.

Detailed, empirical but small-scale study of community practitioner workload and development. Quantitative element uses activity analysis while it qualitatively interviews. Both are used to assess workload and perceptions of staff mix. Anxieties emerged about role change, which were overcome by the bottom-up approach to change management. Key words: acuity, staff mix

Roberts, G. and Anstead, E. (1996) Skill-mix and community profiling in a general practice. British Journal of Community Health Nursing 114: 225–230.

A triangulated approach to assessing and changing the practice skill mix. Health needs assessment, self-managed integrated teams and fund-holding practice issues were combined to review and alter staff mix. Key words: staff mix.

Rodriguez, L. (1994) Skill mix: pick 'n' mix. Health Service Journal 104(5412): 25.

Emphasizes the efficiency and effectiveness effects of properly conducted staff-mix reviews. Key words: staff mix.

Rookes, P.J. (1982) How many health visitors? Nursing Times 78(48): 2043–2045.

Organizationally dated but clear and simple explanation for estimating the size and mix of the health-visiting workforce. Uses activity and caseload data. Key words: dependency, activity and staffing.

Ross, F. (1980a) Primary care in Thameside, Part 1. Nursing Times, Occasional Paper 76(18): 81–83.

Ross, F. (1980b) Primary care in Thameside, Part 2. Nursing Times, Occasional Paper 76(19): 85–87.

Organizationally dated but methodologically valuable small-scale study of one primary health-care team. Examines patient access, referral, dependency, activity and staff mix. Key words: staff mix, dependency, activity.

Rowe, A. and Mackeith, P. (1991) Is evaluation a dirty word? Health Visitor 64: 292–293.

Revisits evaluating efficiency and effectiveness in a health-visiting context. Eschews hard data from process measures in favour of qualitative processes and outcomes. Key words: efficiency and effectiveness.

Rowe, J., Wing, R. and Peters, L. (1995) Working with vulnerable families: the impact on health visitors' workloads. Health Visitor 68: 232–235

Shows that families with greater social and clinical needs receive more targeted health visiting time. Suggests ways highly dependent families can be identified. Includes ample hard data. Key words: dependency and activity.

Royal College of Nursing (1993a) The GP Population Profile. London: RCN.
Royal College of Nursing (1993b) Profiling the General Practice Population. London: RCN.

Explore local health and health-care needs assessment, and the relationship between health care and social care. Clear and succinct accounts. Key word: dependency.

Royal College of Nursing (1994) Public Health: Nursing rises to the challenge. London: RCN.

Short, focused account and guidance for nurses involved in public health work. Sets out the principles and practice of public health from a health needs assessment to planning and implementation angle. Key words: dependency and activity.

Royal College of Nursing (1997) Practice Nursing and Skill-mix. Issues in Nursing and Health 42. London: RCN.

Succinctly sets out the issues surrounding primary health-care team staff mix. Concentrates on practice nursing. Includes useful pointers to assessing and changing staff mix. Key words: staff mix.

Seccombe, I. and Buchan, J. (1993) High anxiety. Health Service Journal, 103(5373): 22–24.

Generates insights into time out, especially sickness-absence data and how they can be used in workforce planning. Key words: time out.

Seccombe, I. and Smith, G. (1997) Taking Part: Registered nurses and the labour market in 1997. Brighton: University of Sussex, IES.

Detailed examination of supply-side workforce planning. Rich in data and analyses. Key words: recruitment and retention.

Seymour, J. (1994) Skill-mix: building a skill-mix team. Health Visitor 67: 105–106.

Anecdotal account of one area's change to include nursery nurses in the workforce. The rationale for and careful approach to change is discussed. Key words: staff mix

Shepherd, M. (1992) Comparing need with resource allocation. Health Visitor 65: 303–306.

Uses caseload analysis to assess and modify workload. Shows how community profiling can spotlight areas of great need and unfair workload among health visitors. Provides insights into the relationship between staffing and workload, noting that there is little correlation between high-risk families and staffing levels. Key word: methods.

Shields, M. and Ward, L. (2001) Improving Nurse Retention in the NHS in England: The impact of job satisfaction on intentions to quit. London: Centre for Economic Policy Research.

Out of print. Key words: recruitment and retention

Sibbald, B., Bojke, C. and Gravelle, H. (2003) National survey of job satisfaction and retirement intentions among GPs in England. British Medical Journal 326: 22–24.

Empirically strong, longitudinal study of GP retention issues. Attitudes between 1997 and 2002 are compared. Job satisfaction fell and intention to stay increased over 5 years. Key word: retention.

Smith, M. (2004) Nursing and healthcare management and policy. Journal of Advanced Nursing 45(1): 17–25.

Detailed, empirical and exploratory study of the present and likely shape of public health visitors' health roles. Examines drivers and restrainers and makes recommendations to strengthen health visitors' public health work. Study was completed before Liberating the Talents. Key word: activity.

Snell, J. (2000a) Workforce planning: fleet of foot. Health Service Journal 110(5692): 26–27.
Snell, J. (2000b) NHS careers: local counsel. Health Service Journal 110(5718): 30–31.

Examine modern supply-side workforce planning issues; some of which influence the demand side. Literature review and interview-based study that compares Department of Health policy with the reality of NHS recruitment and retention of a greying workforce. Underline worrying trends but more importantly what managers can do to alleviate actual and potential problems. Key words: recruitment and retention.

Steele, N., Reading, R. and Allen, C. (2001) An assessment of need for health visiting in general practice populations. Journal of Public Health Medicine 23: 121–128.

Empirically strong quantitative health visitor staffing formula based on four main variables. Application shows that general practice health-visiting establishments were unrelated to need and are largely historical. Key word: staffing.

Stevenson, K., Ion, V., Merry, M. et al. (2003) Primary care: more than words. Health Service Journal 113(5838): 26–28.

Unusual approach to quality assurance involving patients in standard setting and measuring. Raises unusual strengths and weaknesses about service user involvement. Key words: efficiency and effectiveness.

Syson-Nibbs, L. (1997) Skill-mix: skill-mix in a rural health visiting service: a pilot study. Health Visitor 70: 141–143.

Describes a project that widened staff mix by incorporating nursery nurses into health-visiting teams. Strengths and downsides are reported. Key words: staff mix.

Tiesinga, L.J., Halfens, R.J.G., Algera-Osinga, J.T. et al. (1994) The application of a factor evaluating system for community nursing in the Netherlands. Journal of Nursing Management 2: 175–179.

Regression analysis-based method of assessing community patient dependency. Results show that nursing demand can be predicted by a small number of patient and nursing variables. Key word: dependency.

Tobin, T. (2002) Primary care trusts: called to account. Health Service Journal 112(5788): 22–23.

Discusses primary care trusts' financial and management power, which are being jeopardized by a lack of resources, knowledge and skills. Workforce planning is singled out as one weakness. Summarizes the 2001 District Audit and New Organisations, New Responsibilities document (www.district-audit.gov.uk). Key words: staff mix.

Toms, E.C. (1992) Evaluating the quality of patient care in district nursing. Journal of Advanced Nursing 17: 1489–1495.

Literature-based review of community care quality using the quality spiral. Key words: efficiency and effectiveness.

Traynor, M.G. (1995) Job satisfaction and morale in NHS trusts. Nursing Times 91(26): 42–45.
Traynor, M. and Wade, B. (1992a) Feature: I wish I had been an accountant. Health Service Journal 102(5309): 22–24.
Traynor, M. and Wade, B. (1992b) The Development of a Measure of Job Satisfaction for Use in the Monitoring of Morale of the Community Nurses in Four Trusts. London: RCN.
Traynor, M. and Wade, B. (1993) The development of a measure of job satisfaction for use in monitoring the morale of community nurses in four trusts. Journal of Advanced Nursing 18: 127–136.

Examine the interrelationship of job satisfaction, recruitment and retention. Discussions include a breakdown by professional group and underline the main reasons why nurses, for example, are dissatisfied with their jobs. Key words: recruitment and retention.

Trent Health (1991) Caring Principles. General practice guidelines for a quality standard framework. Sheffield: Trent Regional Health Authority.

Outmoded but detailed set of standards and audit questions. Follows the patient through the system. Key words: efficiency and effectiveness.

Triggle, N. (2003) Local care for local people. Health Service Journal 113(5846): 7–8.

Small-scale survey of local health needs from the local authority's and primary care trust's perspective. Priorities were different in the two organizations. Key words: dependency, efficiency and effectiveness.

Tudor-Hart, J. (1971) The inverse care law. Lancet ii: 405–412.

Explores access to and equality of health services. Fairness is questioned when those in most need receive fewer resources and services. Key words: dependency, activity.

Tudor-Hart, J. (1985a) The community debate: When practice isn't perfect. Nursing Times 81(39): 28–29.
Tudor-Hart, J. (1985b) Practice nurse: an underused resource. British Medical Journal 290: 1162–1163.

One GP's view (with some empirical data) of the nature and value of practice nurses. Key words: staff mix.

Turton, P. (1985) The community debate. Jill of all trades? Nursing Times 81(33): 24–25.

Early anecdotal argument for UK public health nurses. Examines their strengths and weaknesses. Key word: activity.

United Kingdom Central Council for Nursing, Midwifery and Health Visiting (1992) The Scope of Professional Practice. London: UKCC.

Sets down the profession's expectations about the nature and value of registered nurse roles. Key word: activity.

Vetter, N.J., Jones, D.A. and Victor, C.R. (1984) Effect of health visitors working with elderly patients in general practice: a randomised controlled trial. British Medical Journal 288: 369–372.

Organizationally and demographically dated study that examines the effects of health visiting services on community elderly patient outcomes. Although mortality was reduced results varied from site to site. Key words: efficiency and effectiveness.

Vetter, N.J., Lewis, P.A. and Ford, D. (1992) Can health visitors prevent fractures in elderly people? British Medical Journal 304: 888–890.

Explores the results of a trial where a large group of community elderly patients were allocated a health visitor, and compared with a control group with no targeted intervention. The number of falls was similar in both groups but 1% more fractures occurred in the intervention group. However, other positive outcomes occurred in the intervention group. Key words: efficiency and effectiveness.

Victor, C.R. and Vetter, N.J. (1984) DNs and the elderly after hospital discharge. Nursing Times, Occasional Paper 80(15): 61–62.

Dated but empirically strong study of the type of elderly patient likely to demand district nurses' time. Patient dependency turns out to be a key variable. Key word: dependency.

Waite, R. (1986) A network for safe staffing. Nursing Times 82(9): 58–60.

Early attempt at setting up a computerized interdisciplinary information and workforce planning system. Key word: establishments.

Walsh, N. and Huntingdon, J. (2000) Testing the pilots. Nursing Times 96(33): 32–33.
Walsh, N., Andre, C., Barnes, M. et al. (2000) New Opportunities for Primary Care? A second year report of first wave PMS pilots in England. Birmingham University: HSMC.
Walsh, N., Roe, B. and Huntingdon, J. (2003) Delivering a different kind of primary care? Nurses working in personal medical services pilots. Journal of Clinical Nursing 12(3): 1–9.

Evaluate some of the first- and second-wave Personal Medical Service pilots. Include important workforce planning and development issues, particularly *Liberating the Talents* and extended roles. Key word: activity

West, M. and Poulton, B. (1997) A failure of function: teamwork in primary health care. Journal of Interprofessional Care 11: 205–216.

Looks at the structures and processes such as the power relationships in primary and community care, and what can be done to reduce the negative elements. Key words: staff mix.

Whitaker, G. (1998) Human resources: monitoring staff turnover: A potential source of cost savings? British Journal of Health Care Management 4(3): 146.

Organizationally dated article that describes a simple but effective and robust demand-side workforce planning method based on timed task and overheads. Key word: establishments.

Whitaker, S.R.M. (1977) A district nurse work analysis. Nursing Times Occasional Paper 79(23): 97–100.

Organizationally and clinically dated article that describes a simple but robust demand-side workforce planning method based on timed task and overheads. Key word: activity.

Whitmore, K., Bax, M. and Jepson, A.M. (1982a) Health services in primary schools: the nurse's roles. Part 1. Nursing Times, Occasional Paper 78(25): 97–100.
Whitmore, K., Bax, M. and Jepson, A.M. (1982b) Health services in primary schools: the nurse's roles. Part 2. Nursing Times, Occasional Paper 78(26): 103–104.

Dated but detailed study of school health services. Robust triangulation is used to gather data about school health services from parents, pupils, teachers and health-care professionals. Provides staffing ratios and other useful (outmoded) data. Substantial recommendations are made. Key words: establishments and activity.

Whyte, E. (1984) Clinical: health begins at school, Nursing Times 80(47): 40–42.

Organizationally dated but valuable study of proactive school nursing based around annual health checks. Includes health needs assessment and population-based staffing establishments. Key word: establishments.

Wiles, R. and Robinson, J. (1994) Teamwork in primary care: the views and experiences of nurses, midwives and health visitors. Journal of Advanced Nursing 20: 324–330.

Qualitative study of perceptions of teamwork and related issues of primary health-care trusts' (PHCTs') members. Highlights the strengths and weaknesses among PHCTs along with what can be done to strengthen primary health-care teams. Key words: staff mix.

Williams, I.E., Greenwell, J. and Groom, L.M. (1992) The care of people over 75-years-old after discharge from hospital: an evaluation of timetabled visiting by health visiting assistants. Journal of Public Health Medicine 14: 138–144.

Detailed randomized controlled trial that measured the processes and outcomes of targeting health-visiting assistants at recently discharged 75 year olds. Although some patient subgroups benefited; there were no differences between the intervention and control groups. Key words: staff mix.

Wilson, A., Pearson, D. and Hassey, A. (2002) Barriers to developing the nurse practitioner role in primary care – the GP perspective. Family Practice 19: 641–646.

Qualitative study exploring GPs' perceptions of nurse practitioners. A surprisingly large number of negative perceptions emerge that sometimes run counter to findings in the literature. Recommendations are made to overcome the barriers. Key words: staff mix.

Wiseman, J. (1975a) Activities and priorities of health visitors – 1. Nursing Times, Occasional Paper 75(24): 97–100.
Wiseman, J. (1975b) Activities and priorities of health visitors – 2. Nursing Times, Occasional Paper 75(25): 101–104.

Look at the rationale behind and some methods of measuring health-visiting services. Organizationally dated but the principles apply. Key word: quality.

Wiseman, J. (1982a) Health visiting – what will be its function in the future? Nursing Times Occasional Paper 78(13): 49–52.
Wiseman, J. (1982b) What health visitors do? Nursing Times Occasional Paper 78(29): 113–116.

Outmoded but comprehensive analysis of pre-Korner activity forms. The nature and purpose of health visiting is compared with their preferred activity. Key word: activity.

Worral, J. and Goldstone, L.A. (1980) A general study of district nursing in Wigan. Nursing Times, Occasional Paper 76(6): 21–26. (See also Goldstone and Worral (1980).)

Early and comprehensive study of pre-Korner community practitioner activity that shows wide variation in the types and times of activities. Recommendations are made to capitalize on these data to improve efficiency and effectiveness. Key word: activity.

Wright, C. (2002) General practice. In for the skill. Health Service Journal 112(5814): 26–27.

Short account of one primary care trust's skill-mix change management process. Understaffed practices were given NVQ level 3 assistants and the effects measured. Key words: staff mix.

Wright, S. (1998) Skill mix in health visiting. Journal of Community Nursing 12(3): 16–18.

Short but comprehensive analysis of primary care staff mix. Concentrates on the implications for health visitors. Key words: staff mix.

Yole, T. and Barrett, A. (2003) In the frame. Health Service Journal 113(5857): 26–27.

Describes a community nursing competency-based framework designed to improve recruitment, retention and career progression among other things. Key words: education and training, recruitment and retention.

Young, C. (1997) District nursing competencies: A Bradford perspective. Leeds University: Nuffield Institute for Health, unpublished dissertation.

Detailed look at the district nurses' role in the context of competencies. Key words: education and training.

# Index